SOUL THERAPY FOR THE WORRIED MIND

STEPS AND STRATEGIES TO OVERCOME PROBLEMS,

BROADEN YOUR HORIZONS, AND LIVE YOUR BODY

INTO A BALANCED LIFE

VINCENT KING

Copyright © 2021 by Vincent King

All rights reserved

The content contained within this book may not be reproduced, duplicated or transmitted without direct written permission from the author or the publisher.

Under no circumstances will any blame or legal responsibility be held against the publisher, or author, for any damages, reparation, or monetary loss due to the information contained within this book, either directly or indirectly.

Legal Notice:

This book is copyright protected. It is only for personal use. You cannot amend, distribute, sell, use, quote or paraphrase any part, or the content within this book, without the consent of the author or publisher.

Disclaimer Notice:

Please note the information contained within this document is for educational and entertainment purposes only. All effort has been executed to present accurate, up to date, reliable, complete information. No warranties of any kind are declared or implied. Readers acknowledge that the author is not engaged in the rendering of legal, financial, medical or professional advice. The content within this book has been derived from various sources. Please consult a licensed professional before attempting any techniques outlined in this book.

By reading this document, the reader agrees that under no circumstances is the author responsible for any losses, direct or indirect, that are incurred as a result of the use of the information contained within this document, including, but not limited to, errors, omissions, or inaccuracies.

Table of Contents

INTRODUCTION 1

CHAPTER 1:
You don't have to worry 3
    ACKNOWLEDGE THE PROBLEM...6
    WHY YOU SHOULD NOT FREAK OUT 8
    HOW CAN I CONTROL MY SITUATION? 11
    HOW NOT TO WORRY ABOUT THINGS AND STOP BEING SAD 13

CHAPTER 2
Life and its challenges 17
    LOSS 18
    FAILURE 21
    SETBACKS 24
    ESTABLISHING MORAL COMPASS 26
    MASTERING YOUR MIND...29
    OVERCOMING YOUR STORY 31

CHAPTER 3
The Ripple Effect..34
    Making Better Decisions 35

CHAPTER 4
Atomic Habits 37

CHAPTER 5
Finding the Beauty in Life..41
    Why It Is Good to Live Life No Matter What 42
    Everything Would Be Fine 46
    Bottom Line..47

CHAPTER 6
Exploring Your Emotional Injuries and Hurts 48
    Causes of Emotional Hurts Injuries and Hurt 49
    Strategies to Avoid Emotional Injuries and Hurt 51

CHAPTER 7
Living A Happy Life 56
    Choosing Happiness in Life 56

CHAPTER 8
Overcoming Obstacles 64
    Importance of Obstacles 65
    Steps to Overcome Obstacles 70
    STEP ONE: ANALYZE THE OBSTACLES 70
    STEP TWO: CHANGE YOUR PERCEPTIONS 73
    STEP THREE: OVERCOME THE OBSTACLES 74
    Using the Power of Motivation 77
    Winning the Influence 79

CHAPTER 9
How to Heal Yourself 81
    Quoting Louise; 83
    ASSUMPTIONS: 85
    BELIEFS: 85
    DENIAL 86
    FEAR 86
    LET YOUR FRIENDS BE 88
    TAKE A LOOK AT YOURSELF 89
    SEE YOUR NEEDS THROUGH REPEATED PATTERNS 90
    BE WILLING TO RELEASE THE NEED 90
    DO NOT PROCRASTINATE 90

DO NOT RESENT THE GOOD OF OTHERS 91

DO NOT CRITICIZE YOURSELF 91

UNDERGO THE PROCESS OF LOVING YOURSELF 93

CHAPTER 10
Rules of Living A Good Life 99

30 Rules of Living a Good Life 100

CONCLUSION 116

About the Author 117

INTRODUCTION

A lot of people believe life is hard. Do you think life is hard too? Well, I do not believe so. Indeed, sometimes, life is good and sometimes, it becomes hard towards us. That still doesn't justify that life is generally hard. Let me tell you about Juliet.

Juliet is a 21-year-old student at one of the prominent universities in the country; she had lost her father and her elder brother to an accident when she was just 7 years old. Her mother had been everything for her while growing up, Juliet had gone through series of crises which were due to stress and anxiety while growing up. She had to withdraw from school because she failed to meet up the emotional and psychological requirements needed to pull school through. Juliet had no other way of coping with all these stresses, so she gave suicide a consideration. She tried taking her own life but narrowly escaped and landed in the hospital. When she got discharged, she was referred to me for guidance; I helped her self-heal with the strategies I have compiled in this book.

She's fine now. If you as her how she feels about life, she'd say "life is truly worth living……"

Now, back to our question. Is life so hard? I'd say, No, life is only fair, although some parts of life may look hard, but it is always balanced up by the good sides of life. And just as Juliet would say, "life is worth living".

Challenges in life are bound to happen, different people deal with different problems in life. In fact, in recent times, a good number of youths have dealt with anxiety and depression without knowing how best to cope with life situations. How do you cope when you are faced with challenges? Recovering from a trauma can be really difficult to deal with. And that is why I have written this book.

This book is going to teach you the easy ways to deal with the hard side of life. So, you do not have to worry about life.

Yes, "you do not have to worry", and that is what we are going to name the first chapter of this book.

CHAPTER 1:
You don't have to worry

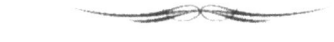

In life, an element of uncertainty is always present therefore making worry inevitable. You are not sure what tomorrow brings, so you worry. You do not know exactly when your problems will be resolved, so you are worried. Worries are part of life. It's even said that "Life is not a bed of roses" which means that bad things are also bound to happen. How do you react when things do not go as expected for you?

No aspect of life is so easy, it is quite okay and normal to worry at some point or the other, however when it becomes a mental habit, it is called "Chronic Worrying". This can seriously affect one's mental and physical health. According to Corrie Ten Boom, "Worry does not empty tomorrow's sorrow, it empties today of its strength." Of course, worrying does not solve and has never solved any problem; it only interferes with your life and makes you get stuck to them. What then is worry?

Worry is simply a feeling of concern about a challenge or a situation. Try to paint a mental picture of you worrying, you would notice that worrying actually makes you uncomfortable and miserable. You might find a good reason to worry but if you find yourself worrying about every little thing every now and then, you would understand that it isn't normal.

Worrying is closely linked with anxiety. In fact, research has shown that a person that worries more often is more likely to die earlier than one that doesn't. While some people may know they worry too much, others may not know. How do I know if I worry too much then? Here are some of the characteristics of worry:

Low self-efficacy
More perceived negative feeling
Hyperactivity
Aggression
More emotional than normal and so on.

Examining yourself based on the above, do you think you worry too much? If you do, follow the solutions recommended here. And if you don't, learn these solutions, they will be useful one day.

Everyone has a problem; even the richest of people have problems. Those celebrities have problems. Your president has problems. Your friends have problems. Your pastor has problems; even your parents have problems. Living in the world, we find ourselves today, there would be challenges. Starting a business and trying to grow it would constitute a lot of worries. Going to college and hoping to get good grades, you have something to think about. Having kids and hoping that you can take care of them, you worry. Having a multinational company, you worry every day about keeping it afloat, especially in the trying times.

What does this mean? It means that life is filled with ups and downs and while you can sit back and worry about these ups and downs, you can choose to see the positive side of things. This is the path to becoming a better person. This is the path to living a life of adventure. This is a path to living because living means overcoming challenges. I repeat, living means overcoming your challenges and becoming better for them.

So, since it is obvious that these challenges are going to come, you should be more concerned about solving the problem rather than worrying about them. In this chapter, I am here to make you understand that you do not need to worry. We would make you understand that life has more meaning than worrying about some things you have no control over. These steps would make you understand more about worrying and how to overcome your worries. Let's go.

Do you know that there are better ways of handling challenges and problems without having to worry? Sounds fascinating right? Well, instead of worrying the whole day long, let's explore how to deal with your challenges better:

(a) Acknowledge the problem
(b) Why you should not freak out
(c) How can I control my situation?
(d) How not to worry about things and stop being sad

ACKNOWLEDGE THE PROBLEM

Do you ever feel like something is wrong with you? Well, you are not alone, almost everyone from time to time wonders if anything is wrong with them, here are some of the signs you should look out for if you feel this way, to be sure there is a problem:

1. An overwhelming feeling
2. Loneliness
3. Physical illness
4. Low self esteem
5. Emotional issues

Note that the first step to take to getting any problem solved is to recognize that a problem actually exists. When some people are faced with a problem, they might ignore it at first; many others may choose to live in denial. It is important to note that challenges are only opportunities to make oneself better. Remember you are the author of your own life and you choose everything that happens in it. Living in denial may be a defense mechanism for some people when they go through stress; they act like such problem does not exist; however, this is not the best way to deal with a challenge as memories would definitely linger no matter how long you try to deny.

Whenever I'm faced with a serious challenge and it feels like it's not going to pass, I make myself understand that there are other people passing through a whole lot more than I am and then I remain calm.

A person that needs to find a solution to a challenge must first assert that there is a challenge, if not, solving it would not work. In fact, it is unethical in many professions to administer help or treatment to a person that doesn't recognize that he or she has a problem.

A lot of us live in self-doubt about our situation. You're worried about something, but anytime the thought of the problem comes to mind, we shove it off, giving it another name or naming another reason why the situation persists.

If you have a problem and you cannot acknowledge it, it remains a problem no matter what you call it. You're worried it could ruin your career, you're worried it could be bad for your relationship, and every time the thought comes to mind, you hide behind the curtain of excuses – you're only postponing the inevitable. But, unfortunately, for some people, it is pride.

The thought of people finding out that they are in this situation gives them the jitters, and rather than acknowledging it to themselves, they bottle it in, and it eats them up. I can relate this to the story of the Instagram celebrity who was depressed because she was alone. Many people seeing how great her life looked on social media, thought she was too good for them.

"The first step in solving a problem is to recognize that it does exist."

Zig Ziglar

This trend continued, and if she had even admitted the problem existed, she would have looked for a solution. But, instead, she kept up appearances till she could no longer do so, committing suicide in the end. Simply put, if pride or any other reason prevents you from telling yourself the truth about your problem, it will end up destroying you.

So, take a pen and a piece of paper and write down that thing causing you to worry; don't worry about telling it to anyone; tell yourself about the problem and acknowledge that it is a problem first. This opens your mind up to the possibilities of searching for a solution and putting it all behind you.

WHY YOU SHOULD NOT FREAK OUT

I use the term "freak out" because many people are paranoid about their situations. The minute they see it as a problem, they want to solve it immediately, and they make panic mistakes. Now that you have recognized a challenge actually exists, it is now up to you to face your fears. This may not seem as easy as it sounds anyways, but you should not be intimidated by these problems. My dad used to tell me that "FEAR" means Fake Experiences Appearing Real. This simply improves my capability to overcome any situation I find myself each time I think about it. Here are a few reasons why you should not allow your problems scare you:

It Does Not Help

Panic never helps. Whenever you panic, you are not thinking with your brain but with your emotions, and this can get the best of you 99% of the time. It's like your brain is offline. When you panic, it is simply your entire being responding to a scenario in which it is unfamiliar. Giving it the space to increase and dominate you only makes you emotional in an unrealistic way, which does not help your situation.

It causes stress

Panic leads to stress – there's no way around it. When you panic, your body releases the stress hormone known as cortisol. Cortisol is like a defense mechanism that the body uses in tough situations, but activating this hormone every time you worry can be detrimental. So, you need to avoid freaking out to prevent this hormone from causing your body any damage.

You are not alone

A lot of people might be overwhelmed by their problems and practically think no one has actually been in their shoes before. The truth actually is that many others have gone or are going through what you might be experiencing today. Thinking about the fact that others might be in this situation as well can make you a little relieved.

The Worst-Case Scenario is not your reality

When you have a disturbing situation, the mind travels a long way looking through the possibilities of how things would turn out, and we look for the worst-case scenario. However, the worst-case scenario is not set in stone. It is not your reality, so you do not need to overthink the situation and plan for a scenario that has not happened. Instead, think of other positive possibilities, ones which would make you less anxious and disturbed.

Every problem has a solution

It is true that problems are real; it is also true that solutions are also real; you only need to discover it. It will only be draining if you should worry about your problems instead of find possible solution to it.

Understand that you can grow from this problem

Every challenge you experience is a chance to grow. For instance, if your business fails, your capacity to overcome this challenge is a big chance to grow. Yes, problems are tough to handle, but when you set yourself up to overcome those problems rather than worry and freak out about them, you have put it behind you. This means that if this happens to surface once again, you have already overcome it before, and you can most certainly do it again, and that is growth.

Problems do not kill, worrying does

My doctor used to say that most people that experience life threatening diseases do not actually die as a result of them but what kills them is the thought of having to live with that disease. This should be enough reason why you should certainly not allow your problems scare you.

There is a lot to be grateful for

While you freak out about your problems, you tend to forget about all the other things you have. You forget about the things you already have. For example, you do not have as much money as you want, and you worry that you would not meet up with your expenses *in the future*. This keeps you from being grateful for most of the things you have now, and with your worried face always there, you lose what you have. You need to balance your thoughts and rewire your brain to see things from a positive perspective because, without it, you are bound to always be worried.

It may become more difficult finding a solution

A lot of people that allow their problems scare them actually take longer in finding a solution to their problem because it only feels like it is impossible to get a solution.

HOW CAN I CONTROL MY SITUATION?

"Control your thoughts. Decide about that which you will think and concentrate upon. You are in charge of your life to the degree you take charge of your thoughts."
Earl Nightingale

Now that you know that freaking out is not the solution to the problem, you need to understand that you have what it takes to overcome your problem and self-heal from all the damage your worrying has caused you.

You just need to soul search deep within yourself and tell yourself, "I can do it." These situations come and go for everyone, and the only ones who are better off are those who see them as an opportunity to grow. Getting to the point you are today is no easy feat and moving on from that problem is not bigger than you.

You just need to wake up in the morning and tell yourself, "I got this." When you do this, you have not only given yourself the power to overcome, you have tipped the balance in your favor, and this is something you can and will do for yourself.

Does it feel like you cannot control your situation? Does everything seem too much for you to handle? Relax, remember you are the author of your own life, if controlling your situation seems really difficult; here is how you can gain control:

Stay calm

One of the easiest and fastest ways to control any situation you find yourself in is by remaining calm. You can stay calm by simply closing your eyes, taking a deep breath and mediating for a few minutes. You can repeat this for a few times till you feel calm enough. It would shock you that you might be able to find out a creative solution to your challenges while trying to remain calm.

Talk to someone

Expressing how you feel can help you get relieved, at least a little bit. It is therapeutic to talk to someone you trust whenever you feel overwhelmed. This can help you stay calm till possible solutions are figured out.

Write down the way you feel

Instead of bottling up your feelings, its best you write them down to let things out of your mind. Once you have written them out, read them out aloud. Also, write down how you hope to overcome the situation and make it a daily routine. This approach works mainly for introverts that find it difficult relating with people. Writing down your goals is important to achieving them; writing down your worries helps you put your worries on paper, which reduces the need to think too much. It is just like emptying your thoughts, freeing your mind in the process. This makes you reassess the situation, and this makes you less anxious about your problems.

Practice positive stress management techniques

Stress is the major reason why people feel overwhelmed, at this point, it is best you practice positive stress management technique to help you control your situation. Positive stress management technique could be as easy as taking a break from work for a five-minute walk or even taking out time to relax and talk with some friends.

HOW NOT TO WORRY ABOUT THINGS AND STOP BEING SAD

Some days, we find it difficult to stop worrying. It does not feel good worrying; it would only make you suffer twice while it does not even stop things from happening. Now that you can now control your situation, it is important that we examine some of the best strategies to keep yourself from worrying:

Stop your online addiction

The world has gone digital, and while there are many positives, a lot of us are addicted. Spending hours upon hours on your social media feeds looking at the picture-perfect lives of others does not do your psyche any good. Many people use social media to escape their problems, and whenever they feel troubled, they get right back at it, streaming away from their problems. If you are an online addict, you need to set the record straight on your online and offline time to better control your life and emotions.

Be Mindful

One of the best strategies to stop yourself from worrying is mindfulness. This involves knowing the thoughts going through your mind and stopping them on their tracks. Being mindful keeps you on top of your thoughts, giving you the chance to filter your thoughts and taking out the negative ones. With a positive mindset attained by being mindful, you disengage from the usual responses you have towards worrying. This gives you a clear mind which is open to the possibilities of solving your challenges as they come. This means more constructive thoughts and less worrying.

Cut yourself some slack

Sometimes, the earnest need to solve every problem immediately can be overwhelming. The specific time does not matter; you are still good as long as you can solve the problem. This is not self-denial; rather, this is you giving your mind the chance to rest from a hostile and difficult situation. If you are excessively scared of a challenge, you overwhelm yourself, making finding a solution almost impossible.

Take Out Time to Meditate

Meditation is a mental practice that helps to soothe your mind and release the anxiety in your brain. Meditation is another practice that leads to a high level of mental consciousness, and what's great about it is that it's not difficult to learn at all. Once you begin and constantly meditate, it becomes a part of you, and your mind becomes powerful enough to overcome your challenges.

Try these as well:

1. Avoid making worrying a mental ability by getting tied with your problem. Instead, focus on getting a solution to your problem. Don't forget we already mentioned that every problem has a solution.
2. Divert your worries into a job to keep your mind away from your problem, if not, it would hurt your present as well as your future.
3. Always try to stay positive no matter how difficult your situation may be.
4. Go for some exercises, this is really helpful in reducing stress
5. See a counselor when the burdens become too much for you to bear.
6. Improve on your interpersonal relationship with others
7. Learn a new skill every time
8. Keep a daily journal on how you feel and how you hope to overcome it
9. Make sure you rest well and follow a good sleeping schedule.

10. Overall, it is best you practice a lot of love even when you do not feel loved, channel your energy into loving others. It would definitely keep worries away.

Bottom Line

You have sole ownership of your life, and you have the power to decide how things go. There are two paths to life – the path of overcomers and those who are defeated. Nobody can make this decision for you but you.

So, you can either choose the path of depression where your worries would get the best of you and your situation, or you can choose to take the steps to self-healing as applied in this chapter. You have all it takes to control your situation, which means that you do not need to freak out for any reason whatsoever.

CHAPTER 2
Life and its challenges

As we said earlier, there is a high level of uncertainty with life. You either choose to enjoy the ride and make the most of everything that comes your way, or you can choose to feel sorry for yourself complaining about everything that comes your way or blaming everyone for your woes. When you choose to feel sorry for yourself, you lose touch with life and what it has to offer, but if you choose to be happy, on the other hand, the challenges help you become a better person, a better version of yourself.

You improve with every passing day, and you always see room for improvement whenever you choose to see your challenges from the standpoint of happiness. You take advantage of the improvements, and you likewise change your levels. In this chapter, we would be taking a look at some of the challenges you would face and overcome on your road to becoming a better person in life.

Sometimes in life, it might feel like you have it all figured out while other times, it might seem as though the world is crashing right in front of you. I personally like this popular saying "When Life gives you lemons, make lemonade out of them" because it keeps me going whenever I am faced with any challenge. It is simply a choice to deal with life challenges or to get drained by them all the time. Whichever one you pick, you should have it in mind that the latter absolutely robs you of the "enjoyments, growth and development" you are supposed to have.

A challenge is basically a new situation that may be difficult and as such requires much effort and determination to overcome. Challenges are not new, from the beginning of the world; different people have been faced with one challenge or the other.

Would you rather love to tell people your story once you become victorious so that they can learn from it or you just want to be pitied? For you to be able to enjoy life to its fullest there are so many life challenges you must learn to overcome some of which are:

i. Loss
ii. Failure
iii. Setbacks
iv. Establishing Moral compass
v. Mastering your mind

LOSS

One of the inevitable events of life is Loss. Loss is simply having something taken away from you, it is called a loss because it is something important. Many people lose things of great importance to them or even someone, this may end up being traumatic to them.

I should tell you about Victor. Victor saw his parents die before his own eyes; they all were making a journey till the driver lost control and bashed into a big pole right in front of the road. Victor was the only survivor in the bus of 11 passengers. It was such a terrible sight for the poor boy. It's been 4 years now but Victor hasn't even gotten past that unfortunate event. Victor's story is quite saddening but death is no respecter of persons, it can happen to anyone at any time, you don't have to wonder why it happened to you and not someone else. That is a clear example of a loss.

Whether you lose a relationship, a job, or a relationship, losing something is part of life. It is inevitable that at some points, you would lose something you love. No matter the circumstances of the loss, it is one of the most difficult things you might have to face. It can be difficult to lose something, but when it happens, it gives you the chance to move forward, reflecting on the things that are most important to you.

Whenever you lose something important to you, it opens you up to a time of self-reflection where you ask yourself, "was this thing of value to me or not?" You also ask yourself what you are willing to do to get what you want later in the future.

When you experience loss, you sit back and reflect on the things that are of value to you. This gives you an understanding of what is of value to you and what is not; at this point, you understand yourself. You understand who you are and your values.

How can I overcome loss? This question is probably ringing in your ears. Of a fact, every individual will lose something at one point or the other. It must happen and the only thing we can try to do is to learn to cope with the loss or try to recover the recoverable. Overcoming loss is not so easy as we often thought, but it is not impossible. It might take a little time, however, if you are in this position, don't fret, here are steps to overcoming losses in a short time:

Be patient with yourself

The first step in overcoming loss is being patient with yourself, you should give yourself time to process and accept all that has taken place. Some people mistake being patient with themselves for living in denial. While healing would occur after being patient with yourself, people that live in denial rarely heal. Try not to remain in this position for such a long time, do not bottle up your feelings and emotions, if you need to cry, then cry! This would help quicken the healing process and make you accept whatever the situation is, faster. Regardless of whatever loss it is, remember "once there is life, there is hope".

Adjust your expectations

Things do not always go as planned all the time and it is only natural to feel very sad about this. You would definitely overcome! Losing a loved one can make you devastated but you only need to adjust your expectations before you completely lose your way. Remember you won't be in this situation for ever, life goes on and you need to go on with life.

Improve your interpersonal relationship with people

Being alone all the time can only make you worry all day long. Even if it feels like you are alone in your situation, you can only make things better by talking to others, sharing your challenges with them. In fact, it is best you talk to someone who has been in the same or similar situation as yourself because this can be quite comforting.

Learn from your experience

Sit back, take a cold drink, and ask yourself what you have learnt from this experience. We say every experience comes with a lesson. I once asked a friend what it felt like losing her legs, she said "Well, nothing lasts forever; it is probably for a reason". I was shocked, who could have thought? She already accepted herself and was ready to move on. Remember every disappointment is a blessing in disguise.

Celebrate Life

If you only focus on what you have lost, then you might be doing yourself more harm than good. It is actually very painful to do so but it can never bring back whatever has been lost. If you lost a loved one, take a moment to think whether your loved one would want you to be sad or happy. Definitely has to be the latter. You are alive and that's a big win, celebrate it, you need to live the moment!

FAILURE

If you were honest with yourself, you would understand that failure is a part of life. The only difference between those who eventually succeed and those who fail is perspective. Those who fail and rise, they see failure as a chance to see things from another perspective. They choose to see failure as a stepping stone to success. Thomas Edison was the inventor of the light bulb, which pioneered many designs today.

He tried about 999 different designs without any success, but the 1000th design brought the results he was looking for, and this made him the renowned scientist he is today. When asked about his failures, he said he did not fail 999 times; rather, he learned 999 different ways not to design the electric bulb. He saw his failures as stepping stones to success, and that was what he achieved.

When you experience failure, you develop empathy and a high level of compassion. You see people in the same situation, and you feel their pain. Understanding how they feel would push you to give advice or help them get better, and this would cause people to feel happy and safe around you.

One life challenge which one must learn to overcome in life is failure. Regardless of how big or small what you have failed is, you might feel shameful or sad, it's only normal. Personally, I feel failure is one of the biggest setbacks to deal with because if not well handled, it can result in depression or even suicide. A wise man once said that failure affords you to try again but better this time. The reason a lot of people feel reluctant to try again after they must have experienced failure is shame and this may be because they were over confident at some point. Have you experienced failure before? Are you finding it difficult to put yourself together and move forward? Here is how you can deal with failure:

Avoid feeling threatened

Many times, people find it hard getting back up when they fail because they feel threatened by failure. Too many people dwell on failure and think that they cannot succeed again after an incident. Replacing negative or threatening feelings with positive ones can help you get over failure faster than you think.

Avoid using bad habits as a defense mechanism

Defense mechanisms are simply a set of behaviors people use to take or separate them from events that are not pleasant, defense mechanisms may reduce anxiety for a while but it does not take it away. One of the most common is Denial. Sometimes, when people go through an unpleasing or a traumatic event, they try to live in denial and pretend it never happened but that does not actually take the hurt away. Other people use bad habits as defense mechanism, for instance, some people eat uncontrollably when they are faced with difficulties, some smoke, some take excess alcohol, etc. Rather than solving the problem, these habits create more problems.

Take responsibility for your failure

Failure is not a disease; therefore, you should not be afraid of taking responsibility for your failure if you want to get over it and become more productive. Keep it in mind that your failure only serves as an experience or a lesson, get the root cause of your failure and deal with it rather than blaming someone else or something for your failure. This will only elongate your healing process.

Read inspiring stories of failures

A lot of people have once gone through failures in life and they eventually turned their failures around into successes. How was this possible? It is only because they stopped dwelling on the past and started focusing on the future. This is by far one of the best strategies in coping with failure. It's completely normal to feel like a failure sometimes, however reading inspiring stories of people that were once failures would make you feel like "yes, someone has actually been in these shoes before and was able to pull through….." have it in mind that if they can do it, you can also do it and let that be a motivational force to doing better.

SETBACKS

Known by many names, "setback" is a part of everyone's journey in life. On your journey to achieving your goals and becoming a better person for yourself, your family, and society, you will experience setbacks. Still, the challenge for most people is understanding the reason for the delay or setback in the first place. You have the opportunity to learn something new. You get to understand what caused you to slow down, and then you have the chance to overcome them and eventually prevent them from happening again. When you overcome your setbacks, you become tough. You develop a mental resilience that allows you to seek solutions that do not compromise your integrity in any way.

Setbacks are situations that slow down one's progress or even regresses one's progress. Nobody plans setbacks, they come up most times when one least expects them and they make one frustrated at the end of the day. People say that if you overcome setbacks, you only become stronger than you were. Well, I agree with that because after I was able to pull through mine, I became stronger. Do you want to know how I pulled through the setbacks I've had? Try these:

Don't panic

It is only very natural to try panicking after one must have experienced a setback, this is due to fear, for instance, a person who has lost a job and has the sole responsibility of feeding a family of four would definitely want to panic. However, avoiding panic would help you pull through setbacks faster and stand on your feet to face those setbacks.

Expect the worst

Most entrepreneurs and business men are risk takers and as such, they have higher chances of dealing with setbacks at one point or the other. If you were in the position of losing a huge amount of money, how would you react? Do you know what these people do? They expect the worst! Yes, they sit down to ask themselves the worst that could happen if they their money. The trick is, nothing surprises you anymore when you do this, whatever comes with the day, you're already prepared for it. Instead of worrying about what the day would bring, you are calm with plans on how to cope with them.

Eat and rest well

Getting a good amount of rest can help in improving your mood as well as your energy. Experts have said that a good amount of sleep shouldn't be less than seven hours a day, this means that if you sleep for less than 7 hours a day, you have not had a good rest. Also, we know the saying "You are what you eat ". This simply implies that our physical and emotional well being is manifested by what we eat. Some specific meal can help reduce feeling of depression.

Don't live in the past

The past is simply before you had any setback whatsoever. You would be living in a fool's paradise if you keep dwelling on whatever you had in the past. Instead, focus on developing yourself better each day. You can do this by setting a time range for yourself, for example, 2 weeks, 1 month, 1 year and so on. Then, keep a journal to track and record your growth during this period. Some time ago, I experienced a major setback in my business. I made sure I learnt a new trade every two weeks just to develop myself and keep my mental health intact. And this helped me to be a better person.

ESTABLISHING MORAL COMPASS

Have you ever rejected a job regardless its pay because it isn't legitimate? Well, I have, because I have clearly established my moral compass. Early in life, we all establish our moral compass which influences our decision making. No two persons have the same moral compass, this means that every moral compass established is peculiar to every individual.

What then is moral compass? A set of fine-tuned values (core) that help influence your decision making all through your life. Sadly, many people cannot pin point what their core values are. Generally, your moral compass should not only be good to you but also the society at large. Many people make decisions that may be fair to them without considering if it is fair to the society. Also, establishing a moral compass is not just enough, what is enough is living by what you have set to be your core values.

Does having a moral compass stop you from having challenges in life? The answer is No, many challenges come unexpectedly. What a moral compass does is that it only helps you in managing your challenges in the sense that it places a balance between your emotions and your sense of reasoning. It makes you make rational decisions even when you may experience loss, failure or setbacks.

Understanding the difference between right and wrong is another life challenge you would experience. You might have one mindset today and then another tomorrow because you have the right to change your mind at any point. Changing your mind is your right and where you stand is your responsibility, and your choice can help frame you into a better person as you try achieving your goals.

Your beliefs and values determine your actions, and examining them would help you grow and become a better person. If at some points, you get to find out that your goals and beliefs are not in alignment with your goals, then you can change them.

Once you find out that your moral compass does not align with your goals, you can change them and point yourself in the right direction; one which would serve you well on your journey to success.

Have you been able to fine tune your moral compass? Are you confused on what to do? Here is how you can fine tune your moral compass:

Get a grip of what you consider to be moral

Getting a grip of what you consider to be moral will help you in fine tuning your moral compass. It is important to note that what a person considers to be moral may be quite different from what you feel moral should be, although, you can learn from others.

Make sure your values are similar to your behavior

You cannot be a dishonest person while establishing honesty as your value, it just wouldn't work for you, take a seat, study yourself. If you need to change some of your attitude that would hinder making a great moral compass, then do. You can simply write down a list of what you want to be your moral value and work on your behavior so that they both work simultaneously and not against each other.

Never betray yourself

This may sound easier than actually keeping to it. No matter how little, make sure you do not sell your integrity for anything. You already know your compass, stand your ground on it, be firm even when you are offered money or material things. Once you have a good moral compass, you're more likely to have more positive outcomes.

Respect other people's boundaries

If you want others to respect your boundaries, then you shouldn't over step others' boundaries. It is a compass because there are boundaries. People tend to overstep people's boundaries by not regarding their values because they are not similar to theirs.

Once these principles are followed religiously, you would definitely have a great moral compass that fits in your behavior that allows you improve productivity and also reduce damage(s).

MASTERING YOUR MIND

Your mind is an important part of your success journey, and it can be your best friend or your worst enemy, depending on whether you master it or make it your master. When you have a situation, your mind brings up all kinds of negative thoughts and ideas, and for those who have not mastered their mind, it takes over.

Mastering your mind is a big challenge because your mind controls your perspective, and it determines the way you interact with the world around you. It takes a lot of time and practice to master your mind. This means that it would take a lot of hard work to master your emotions, but if you take it one step at a time, you will end up winning the battle over the control of your mind.

This is a challenge you have to take seriously because if you have a mind filled with negativity and let this negativity rule over you and your actions, becoming a better person will be hard. Some of the best ways to master your mind are meditation, prayer, journaling, and self-reflection.

For the creation of a good life, we know very well that the mind is a very powerful tool, however, if you do not manage it properly, it can turn to be the most destructive weapon in your life. No doubt, our mind definitely tampers with what we interpret to be reality. According to research, an average man has more than 60,000 thoughts daily imagine how that would be a waste of time if the thoughts are not even productive. Here is what you need to do to properly master your mind:

Pay more attention to positive mental thoughts

We have said earlier that it is only natural to worry about things. We actually find ourselves worrying about negative things most times, the earlier you realize that you cannot do much by merely thinking about what happens to you, the better. We however cannot stop ourselves from having negative thoughts but when we pay more attention to positive thoughts, it helps us master our mind more.

Make use of meditation

Meditation is an ancient technique to mastering your mind. Our fathers used it. Who said it no longer works? Of course, it does. The trick meditation does is that it calms your brain and relieves it of stress. Do you know that when your mind isn't stressed, you have more chances of having positive thoughts? Whenever you have too much going on in your mind, practice meditation.

Forget the past, Focus on the future

One great torture you can do to your self is ruminating over the past for a long time. "What if I had done it better? I shouldn't have done this or that...." No, don't do that. These events are already beyond your control. Focus on how you can make it better in the future. Unless you push the past aside, it is impossible to master your own mind.

Mastering your mind may take a while, it does not just happen in a moment. Also, keep in mind that it is much easier and less expensive managing a healthy mind than an unhealthy one.

OVERCOMING YOUR STORY

Your story is what it is; your story but does not have the power to determine where you are headed except you give it the power to overcome you. Most of the richest people in the society today have a story to tell. The only difference between those who achieve success and those who do not is their capacity to overcome those stories.

If you do not overcome your story, you would feel like the placement you find yourself cannot be overcome, which sinks you further into depression, sadness, and a lack of achievement. Overcoming your story requires you to be intentional and aware of yourself, letting go of the negative energy and climbing on the ladder of positivity.

This would not only help you become successful, but it would also encourage others to overcome their stories and become better individuals in the end. In addition, this means that you can write your own story for yourself and be in total control of your life. This would cause you to panic less and be in much more control of your situations and circumstances.

Every successful person in life has a story to tell, they were not just born successful, many of them burnt their fingers to be where they are today. One major difference between a successful person and an unsuccessful one is that the former overcame their story. Don't you want to overcome your story too? Let's explore how you can turn your story around.

First, get rid of fear! Fear is the reason why you have not gotten a better version of yourself. I would be lying if I said you can stop yourself from being afraid, it is only very natural to be afraid of some situations but what I mean is that whenever fear tries to get between you and your dreams, ignore it. Remember I said earlier that to me, fear means fake experiences appearing real. It helps me overcome fear all the time when I remember "everything going on in my head is not real." Take a glass of water whenever you feel nervous. It helps to calm your nerves.

Next, you need to get rid of the fear of failure. People are often scared of competing or trying again because of the fear of failure. Not every action you take will be successful, don't always expect that. What failure does is that it gives room for improvement. I always tell myself that I cannot fail what I've failed before simply because I have learnt from my mistakes.

Finally, this point is a very crucial one as people may not see it as a barrier to overcoming one's story but I do. You need to get over the fear of success. Many people think success is just for extraordinary people. They don't think they deserve to be successful as well. You don't have to suppress your gift because you feel you don't deserve it. Every one of us deserve good things. Now it's up to you to turn your story around!

Bottom Line

The common denominator in life is challenges. You would face these six challenges no matter what you do and where you are on your road to achieving success. The only difference between you and those who fail is that you have the information, and this information would help you self-reflect and permit you to re-evaluate what you believe and what you stand for in life. This takes away the negativity and gives you the power to self-heal

CHAPTER 3
The Ripple Effect

In a bid to make you understand the importance of your decision to self-healing or not, we have decided to take a look at the ripple effects of your decisions. When a lot of us make decisions, we fail to understand the consequences of such actions – much of which spans far beyond our control. When we have a decision to make, our major focus is on the challenges at hand, and most of the time, we miss the bigger picture. Our priorities are based on the things we want to achieve now, not knowing that the decision has bigger consequences.

You need to understand that every choice has bigger and lasting consequences beyond the small objective you wish to achieve. Think of it like dipping your finger into still water. It seems like a small and inanimate action, but in truth, it goes far beyond the small spot affected by the finger dip. This means that each decision you make can affect you in unimaginable ways and likewise affect those around you, including your children, friends, family, and those who believe in you.

Knowing how important this is, you owe it to yourself and those around you to think about the consequences of your actions. You owe it to yourself and those sets of people to increase your level of understanding about your actions and understand the importance of your choices and the resulting action.

Making Better Decisions

To make better decisions, we would be taking a look at three important steps that would help you make better decisions with ripple effects that would lead to positive ripple effects.

1. **Take time to focus**: making a decision is not an easy task, and it can be much more difficult when there are numerous outcomes to consider. Some decisions are difficult to handle sometimes, and when faced with the call, we make impulsive decisions. Some other times, we avoid making decisions altogether, which is still not a good decision. One of the most confident decisions based on your thoughts after taking some time off to think about the situation. You simply have to clear your mind, concentrate and think about the possibilities your actions can lead to. Most importantly, think about the reason for deciding the first place and why the decision matters.
2. **Listen to others**: while you are a special person with a distinctive personality, no man is an island. When necessary, you can share your thoughts with someone you respect. This allows someone to share their thoughts and perspective with you, giving you the chance to see things from their

perspective. This does not mean you have to take everything you are given; rather, you can be selective with the information, make use of what you feel is important, and leave the rest.

3. **What next**: this is a technique that helps you move forward in a bid to solve the problem rather than trying to look back to see the root cause of the problem in the first place. This helps you count the endless possibilities available to you and the scenarios that can occur due to these scenarios. When you sit back and ask yourself, "What Next," you find your mind searching for the way forward. This is an important technique because it helps you map out different possibilities with the possible outcomes from these decisions.

You need to understand that no matter how much we try; some decisions might not go our way with our emotions getting the best of us. At this point, we find ourselves worrying unnecessarily and getting depressed over our situations. However, when this happens, it is important to sit back and reflect on the situation because the ripple effect of these decisions or inaction spans far beyond our control.

The one certain fact is that not everything would go your way every time, as we highlighted in chapter 2, but what you do after a failure or setback determines whether you would self-heal and become a better version of yourself or otherwise. Challenge yourself to make good decisions. Challenge yourself to make decisions with positive ripple effects. Challenge yourself to make an impact for you and your tomorrow because it is worth it.

CHAPTER 4
Atomic Habits

In essence, if we want to direct our lives, we must control our consistent actions. It's not what we do once in a while that shapes our lives, but what we do consistently.

Tony Robbins

Another important part of your journey to self-healing is your habits. Habits help move you to a point where you are happy. It helps you snap out of unhappy situations, and it helps you improve your life daily. An atomic habit is a routine that is small and easy to do but has incredible power to change your life.

When it comes to being happy, you need to adopt these small atomic habits, which are easily adapted but get you great results in the end. Even with bad events in the past, you find it easy to heal and make better decisions in the future. Here are some of the simplest atomic habits that can guarantee happiness for you and cause you to be cheerful even in difficult situations.

Smile

As small as a smile is, it has a lot of power. We often smile when we are happy but what you never knew is that when you smile, your brain releases dopamine, which causes you to be happier than before. This is not a call for you to keep on walking around with a fake smile, rather a cause to see a reason to smile even in bad times. When you can do this, your mind can look for solutions.

Be Grateful

Being grateful for the things you have can be a big mood booster improving your sense of hope and happiness. You start your day by recognizing the things you are grateful for. This can be done anywhere and anytime of the day. As your day proceeds, even when you face difficulties, try to think about your life's pleasant parts, which bring you a high level of happiness. Think about the good thing you have done for others which gives you joy and resonates with them. They make you understand all you have rather than focusing on what you do not have.

Compliment others

Giving a compliment to others is an act of kindness that improves your level of happiness. The compliment not only makes someone else happy, but it also makes you happy. Make it a habit to compliment someone at home or work every day, and you would be surprised about how good it makes you feel. Always make sure your compliment is respectful to help make sure that result is not defeated.

Get Enough Sleep

It might look like you do not need sleep, but you need it more than you know. Modern society makes sleep look like something less important, but it is more important than you think. To get enough sleep, you need to make a functional sleep routine that would allow you to sleep and work as much as you would like.

Breathe Deeply

When you're tense and unhappy about something, you feel like you just might lose it. Instead of letting your situation get the best of you, take a deep breath and calm yourself down. This process involves closing your eyes, taking slow and deep breaths through your nose, and then repeating the process until you feel perfectly calm. If you find it hard to take deep breaths, try counting while you breathe for better focus.

See a Friend

As humans, we are social beings, and having people around us can make difficult situations less complicated. When it comes to seeing a friend, think of those people who cause you to laugh anytime you see them and take time out to visit them. This practice keeps you talking, and you get less overwhelmed by your situations.

Bottom Line

Atomic habits are small habits that bring big results, and these are the best atomic habits you can start today. These habits brighten your day and give you reasons to smile even when the going gets tough. They might seem inanimate and small initially, but they yield tangible results in the long run.

CHAPTER 5
Finding the Beauty in Life

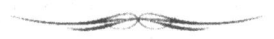

"I can only note that the past is beautiful because one never realizes an emotion at the time. It expands later, and thus we don't have complete emotions about the present, only about the past."
Virginia Woolf

Talking about self-healing and living a happy life, we look to cover another important chapter which I call finding the beauty in life. Humans are very characteristic beings who often find routines and use these routines to get through the day. These routines form our personalities, and we make them a part of who we are.

However, we get tired of these routines at some point, it makes no difference anymore, and we begin to miss the beautiful moments each day carries. We sometimes do not recognize that we have pushed ourselves to the point that we are no longer present in our day, and without this, you fail to see the beauty that comes with each day. Here are some facts you need to know.

Why It Is Good to Live Life No Matter What

Here are some of the reasons you need to live life to the fullest by finding the beauty in life:

You Cannot Be Perfect

If you want to see the beauty in life, you need to understand that you are not and would never be perfect. Even those people you look up to sometimes lose touch of their razor-like focus now and then. There are certain times of the day that feel less important than others and, in these times, you find yourself shifting focus to things that are more important than what you are currently doing. While many people look for different ways to concentrate and focus, you should try seeing the beauty that life has to offer you.

You Can Find the Beauty

Everything is beautiful if you look at it the right way. However, if you are a lover of art like myself, you will notice that even the worst of objects have something unique about them, something which cannot be replicated in any way. These days, the challenge with us is that we choose to overlook this beauty around us even though it is pretty simple.

Seeing the beauty in anything is simple. You just need to look at it from another perspective. For example, if you pass by an old house around your home, you need to take time to see it from a vintage perspective, and you would fully appreciate the beauty the house carries.

You can See the Beauty All Around Us

Once you open yourself up to the possibility of beauty being everywhere, your mind opens up, and you suddenly get to see the things you never got to see before. Seeing beauty everywhere makes you see the beauty in what you have, and it would help you cherish what you have.

The Way You See Beauty Changes

When you see the beauty in the things around you, the way, you see beauty changes. You might have thought your home was not looking great, but all of a sudden, you begin to see the value in what you have. You see the colors feel the texture, and you know you have got something good going on for you.

Everything Becomes More Enjoyable

When you see the beauty in everything and truly appreciate life, you get to enjoy everything that comes your way. Rather than focusing on something which takes away the fun and beauty in it, you see the beauty in it just the way it is. When you turn your attention away from the imperfections to the good side of things, you see the wonderful qualities in everything you see.

You are Present with Your Perspectives

Finally, seeing beauty all around you is about paying attention to your emotions and thoughts in the now. Think of it for a moment; if you are angry, you will see things that would get you angrier. However, you have the power to change this because if you can see the beauty in anything, you get reminded about how wonderful the world is with you in it.

Your life is great; you just don't realize it

Another thing that makes you see the beauty in life is appreciating your own life. The world has gone digital, and with the digital nature of the world today, we compare our lives with that of others, which robs us of the beauty in your own life. Forget everything we have said so far; if you do not see the beauty in your own life, then nothing can ever have meaning to you.

Not everything that glitters is gold, and while you would be better off in someone else's shoes, you do not know what they are going through irrespective of how good things look. Simply put, you have the best life, and until you see it that way, you would struggle with life. Here are some of the reasons why your life is already great:

You are alive

Think of it for a moment, why are you alive in the first place? It must be for a reason, isn't it? So why would you think that your life is not worth something? If you have something and it is not worth anything, you throw it away.

So, if you were not worth anything, you would not be alive today. You have something to give this world, and until you see your value, you would feel you are worth nothing, and this is almost the same as not living at all.

You have enough time

Whenever you achieve anything, you need to understand that it is the right time. We see many people achieving their goals at the age of 50, 60, and even 70, and they feel happy about themselves. Why is that? Because they believe that until the game is over, it is not over.

Even with their setbacks, they believed they still had enough time to achieve what they wanted, and they eventually did. But, when you look at others and see how much they have achieved, and you look down on yourself for not achieving that much within that period, you put a stop to what you can achieve. So, you need to understand that you have enough time to do what you would love to achieve. The minute you cut your time short, you have already lost, and the essence of your life is lost eventually.

Opportunities are Coming Your Way

Everyone has opportunities; practically everyone. The only difference between those who win and those who lose is their capacity to see the opportunities. Opportunities do not always look like opportunities when they come, and only those who can truly see those opportunities would win. Those who never get opportunities are those who do not know how to unravel the ones that come their way. They complain a lot about not getting them, not knowing how much they have already lost. So, think hard. A lot of opportunities must have come your way; the question is: did you make use of them? So, opportunities are always coming, and capitalizing on them would certainly add meaning to your life.

You can choose what you want to do

Having a choice is great, and the world is designed in such a way that you have the power to choose your path. Whether it is your career, your relationship, or your goals, it's all up to you to decide the direction of your life, and believe me when I say it is great that we can all make decisions for ourselves.

If you do not know how great it is making your decisions, then put someone in charge of making your decisions for you, and you would see the beauty in your life. For the mere fact that you can look back at your life and say to yourself, "I lived as I believe," you know that your glory and failures are outcomes you can own up to and not blame anyone for.

You are Loved

Except you choose to be alone, there is always someone somewhere who would always love you for who you are, and that is the truth. Love is a beautiful thing, a marvel in the world, and you have that love. Yes, you might have lost someone, broken up a friendship, or ended things abruptly in a relationship, but someone somewhere is always showing you that they love and care for you, and this is something worth living for. So, think about it. You have someone who cares deeply for you, and that shows the value your life holds.

Everything Would Be Fine

We all experience ups and downs, and although it can be tough, it also defines our stories. So many of the beautiful life stories we have heard have enough essence when we see what people have passed through. The only thing that helps people overcome their problems is the thought that everything would still be fine in the end. So, your life is great. Everything would be fine in the end, and all you need to do is believe. Believe that you can only get stronger from this point, and you would eventually overcome everything you are passing through.

Bottom Line

Life is beautiful; it just takes you opening your eyes to see it. There are countless reasons why life is beautiful, and those who can see it would experience it. First, realize that your life is great, and then doors would begin to open to you. Think of your belief as the key to the endless possibilities in life. If you do not turn the key to belief, the door of happiness would never be opened. The key is in your hands; you just have to use it.

CHAPTER 6
Exploring Your Emotional Injuries and Hurts

Emotional injuries and hurt are the types of pain that come from non-physical sources. Most of the time, these emotional pains come as a result of the action of others, while some other times as a result of loss or grief. Irrespective of the cause of the emotional pain, it can be intense most of the time, spanning other aspects of your life. It can also prevent you from self-healing, which is why you need to make sure you treat these emotional challenges right from the root. While many people take physical pain more seriously, emotional pains are more complicated pains should not be taken with levity. Here are some of the symptoms of emotional pains:

- Shame

- Worthlessness

- Depression

- Grief

- Panic

- Negative emotions

- Deep sadness

- Rage

- Strong distress

- Loneliness

Sometimes, these emotional injuries and hurt become physical to the point that it begins to disrupt all other aspects of your life and your overall ability to function.

Causes of Emotional Hurts Injuries and Hurt

There are a couple of reasons why people face emotional hurts and injuries, and most of the time, they interfere with everything you hold dear, which can be bad for everything you do. Here are some of the major causes of these hurts and injuries

Sadness

Sadness is a feeling practically everyone has experienced at some point in life due to disappointment or loss but what's worse about it is that it does not leave the mind on time and develops to other conditions like depression which impacts everything about you.

Anger

Anger is something we all feel, like a basic part of being human. When you feel angry, you feel the tension in your muscles and causes a rush of adrenaline. This can come in handy when you need it sometimes, but some other times, it can be consequential, especially the resulting actions.

Guilt or shame

The feeling of shame and guilt is a weighty feeling carried everywhere about something bad done. It can also be consequential in the long run.

Anxiety

Just as we pointed out with anger, anxiety also causes an adrenaline rush, preventing anyone from feeling the need to relax. There are numerous reasons why anxiety happens, and it can lead to substance abuse.

How to Manage Emotional Injuries?

One of the first strategies you can use to keep your mind and emotions healthy is the proper management of your emotional injuries and hurt. Here are some of the important strategies that can help you get your emotions right on track:

Practice Mindfulness

When you are emotionally hurt, you experience it physically. You have this sort of heaviness in your stomach, and it often gives you a headache. We sometimes try to escape this feeling, but it becomes more and more overwhelming. The practice of mindfulness helps you notice how you feel and gives you a sense of how to lessen your pains.

Use Many Distractions

We have always been told that every emotion we feel has to be let out or express in another way. This has a certain sense of truth to it but sometimes very unhealthy. We sometimes try to dig deeper than is necessary, and this yields bad results.

A better way to handle situations is to distract yourself with things that can lessen your emotional pains. A simple example is having fun activities with friends.

Set Out Time to Think

Suppose you find your emotional hurt excessively painful. In that case, if you find that distracting yourself does not also work for you, you need to set out a certain time to think about the situation where you can ponder on certain solutions. Then, once you are done, you can relate this to a close friend – someone who is not judgmental – for some friendly advice and some distractions as well.

Meditate

When it comes to your emotions, meditation is one of the best management techniques. Meditation takes your thoughts and helps you positively redirect them. This would help take out most of the stress in your mind, and it works long-term.

Strategies to Avoid Emotional Injuries and Hurt

While managing your emotional injuries and hurt is great, you can also avoid some of them. These avoidance techniques help you understand your emotions, what to expect from those emotions, and how to avoid them. These strategies work for everyone and can be used anywhere and anytime.

Be prepared for it

I know what you're thinking; there are some things we cannot prepare for, and expecting you to prepare is like asking you to predict what would happen throughout the day. However, one thing you can do is improve your emotional intelligence. Emotional intelligence allows you to understand the unpredictability of life and how to handle them.

It gives you a certain level of grit which helps you shift your mind and focus away from the difficulty of the situation to the positivity that comes from the situation. Some people might term you as someone without emotions, but instead, this is you guarding your mind against any mental difficulties that might hurt you.

Think Ahead

Whenever you are faced with a situation that would hurt you emotionally, you need to ponder what has happened and what could happen, and you would see that things are not as bad as they seem. An example is losing your job.

Whenever this happens, it can be difficult for anyone to handle, and while it can be devastating for some people, those who can think ahead would see it as a chance to get another job. A chance to visit somewhere new, a chance to relax, and open their minds to new possibilities. With this mindset, you would face difficulties somehow, and you would likewise not be hurt as much.

Boosting Your Energy

Another important consideration when it comes to exploring your emotional hurt and injuries is boosting your energy. This is more physical because they help to prevent your body from being vulnerable to emotional hurt. Here are some of the best ways to boost your energy:

Control Your Stress Levels

Stressful emotions drain you of your energy, and this is something you have to learn how to control. You can use numerous methods to reduce your stress levels, like talking to a friend, taking a walk, or watching a movie.

Lighten your load

Another reason why you lack the energy levels you need to overcome your emotional stress because you stress yourself excessively. You overwork yourself, and whenever you are emotionally stressed, your body would react the wrong way. If necessary, consider asking for help when you feel overworked.

Exercise your Body

Another thing that keeps your body and emotions in check is exercising. Exercising helps your body burn calories and move oxygen throughout the body. It also increases your dopamine levels, which means you are much happier than you usually used to be before the exercise. It also helps your mood, which is of great importance when it comes to emotional management.

Eat Good Food

Good foods with low glycemic indexes like vegetables, nuts, and oils help improve your bodily functions and mental capacity. This means that whenever your body is faced with a mental battle, it has the right nutrients for these emotions off.

Drink Enough Water

Water is an important part of life because it gives your body the necessary fluids to function properly. With these fluids readily available to you in your system, you would not be overwhelmed by your emotions.

Use Caffeine Wisely

As much as caffeine helps your body and mind stay sharp, too much of it can leave you emotionally vulnerable. On the other hand, when you sharpen your mind with coffee, you feel high energy to help you in emotionally sensitive times.

Bottom Line

Whenever you are emotionally hurt and injured, it can be hard to self-heal. It can be hard to overcome emotional stress. Without the capacity to overcome this emotional stress, we sometimes feel overwhelmed, and it gets the best of us, leading us to make irrational decisions.

This chapter explores the various aspects of emotional hurt and how you can manage or avoid them. We have pointed out some of the best ways to manage and avoid emotional hurt, and it would be very beneficial on your journey towards becoming a better person.

CHAPTER 7
Living A Happy Life

Choosing Happiness in Life

Some years back, I was in college. I used to top the class as I found studying interesting and I picked so much interest in it. As a matter of fact, I studied as though my life depended on it. actually, as at then, I thought my life really depended on it. to crown my efforts, I had the best results and I was proud of myself as much as my parents were proud of me. Everything went well 360 degrees for me. My family was doing fine. My friends were cool and supportive. I was financially buoyant too. Everything was fine until I lost my dad.

My dad was the finance pillar of the family. He was my gist partner. But suddenly, I lost him. Gradually, I started losing focus in class, I plunged into isolation, I started preferring to be lonely. Before I knew it, I couldn't maintain my academic feat, and everything turned direct opposite. At this point, I had two options, whether to be sad or to be happy.

If it was you, what would you have chosen?

I took happiness and if you ever fall in that position, please choose happiness.

People do say "happiness is free" and "happiness is relative". This simply means that what makes you happy may make someone else sad. For example, while getting an iPhone 11 pro max may make me sad, getting the same phone will most likely make someone who used to use iPhone 12 sad. So, many times, we all have the chance to be sad or happy with some happenings in our lives. What I am simply saying is that, in cases like this, choose happiness.

Having a life that you desire goes beyond just making choices that will boost your finance, health or even career. Above all, there is one aim we all are after, and that aim is happiness. We all want to be happy whether we are rich or poor, healthy or unhealthy, tall or short.

Who does not want to be happy? I do want to, and you also want to. Inasmuch as no one should force us to choose happiness, I have decided to show you how to and why you need to choose happiness.

You must note that choosing happiness does not mean that you should just click your heels together a couple of times as you desire to go to a happy place. The secret of happiness is not just in making the right choice, but it is in learning to choose right and to choose well.

One of the best ways to destroy every form of unhappiness and depression in your heart that makes it difficult for you to heal is living a life of happiness. I'm sure that you have come across some individuals with whom it feels like nothing can take away their joy. However, they have found the secret to healing from any form of hurt or emotional pain, living a happy life.

If you are unhappy for some reason, it's not worth it. You owe it to yourself to be happy. Moreover, only those who know how to live happily can overcome situations they find themselves in. Here are some of the easiest ways to attract happiness wherever you go and with whatever you do. It does not matter whatever you have passed through; you can always heal, especially when you are committed to living a happy life.

Be committed to being happy

If you truly want to be happy, you truly have to be committed to being happy. When you set goals, you would experience setbacks, and these setbacks can make it difficult for anyone to see the light at the end of the tunnel. However, for those who have chosen to be happy and have committed themselves to be that way, things eventually work out. For example, imagine someone having his life's work burnt to the ground; the first expression should be sadness, but instead, he looks at his son and says to him; tomorrow we start building again, and he does it with a smile on his face as well. This shows how committed he was to be happy, and this commitment helped him build things right back up and even better.

Understand that people love you and not your success

I have seen a lot of men go bankrupt and rise back up and even better. This is because they understand that those things are just material. If they were concerned about what people would think about them losing their fortunes, they would probably die from the depression. You are a lovely person, and those who care about you do so because you are a lovely person and not because you have achieved anything. If you have this in mind, you would not be bothered about what people would think about your situation.

Be grateful for everything

If you take a clear look at what you go through every day, the fact that you are still alive is enough to be grateful for. I read a book where the author clearly stated that if you were to walk a mile in the shoes of others, you admire so much, you would cherish what you have, and it is true. If you can see the value and essence of what you have and see reasons to be grateful for it, then you would be happy. You have to know that only those who are truly grateful for what they have now qualified for the next blessings coming their way.

Take Action

Inaction and laziness reduce your belief in what you can and would accomplish in life. You know what you carry, and when you are not doing anything about it, you feel sad, feel depressed, and tired of your existence. On the other hand, when you take action, you believe in yourself and what you can accomplish with your baby steps. Those steps – as small as they are – can take you to greater heights of life, and this makes you happy. Also, take action to help others become happy, and just as we talked about the ripple effect, it would come back to you in ways you never imagined possible.

Understand that money cannot buy happiness

We all like to have money. I mean, if there's anyone who does not want money, you can send it to me, and I'll be happy. Yes, money is important, but it cannot buy you happiness. So, if you think the wealth you are gathering can bring you happiness, you need to guess again. Other things like your passion, family, friends, people, country give people happiness depending on who you are, and the earlier you understand this, the better.

Avoid taking rejection personally

Rejection is a part of life. It happens to the best of us at some point or the other, but you have got to understand that being rejected is not a verdict. It is not a mark of shame placed on your forehead, and you have to avoid wearing it that way. Instead, for every rejection, you need to learn something and make the required changes. For example, the girls always rejected me back in high school because I never took grooming seriously.

It affected my self-esteem so much that I was not happy being around girls. When I understood this in college after a few rejections, I took my grooming seriously, and you know the rest of the story. I got rejected sometimes, but I also got some girls. I learned that not everyone could like you, which is their loss; you just have to look at yourself and make changes without losing your happiness. It cost me a lot of happiness in high school; I'm glad I learned to be happy.

Improve your social skills

Data shows that most people who are unhappy at work or in social gatherings have poor social skills, which causes them to get rejected a lot. Instead of letting this derail you, you can improve your social skills and become more socially inclined. This would improve how you interact and prevent socially awkward situations where you freeze and find it hard to say anything.

Travel to somewhere new

As we said previously, we are bound to get bored about some things at some point, and we feel like life has become more programmed than it is enjoyable. For you to lighten up, you need to travel to somewhere new at some point in the year or another. When you travel, you see and feel something new, and this can breathe life into your boring and programmed life, as you call it. It also helps to create memories, many of which you can reminisce on and smile. You can also look at those pictures and be happy knowing that your next journey is coming pretty soon.

Avoid Multitasking

Your mind is a supercomputer, but even supercomputers get burnt out at some point or the other. One of the best ways you overburden your mind is by multitasking, doing about five things simultaneously, which can cause your mind to be unsettled and overly tasked. So, for everything you want to do, a better idea would be to plan. Plan everything from the first to the last and take out time to rest in between tasks to prevent the same thing from happening over again.

Embrace the mindset of growth

Knowing that you are growing through the rough patches can keep you going, but that is if you know you are growing. For whenever you fail, you need to tell yourself that you are not a failure; rather, you are someone who is passing through a phase, one which you would be better off for when you eventually overcome your troubles. With the growth mindset, you can never be put down; instead, you keep growing stronger and stronger with each day and each challenge that comes your way.

Do not hold grudges

When we hold grudges with someone else, we are not hurting them but ourselves. We have them in mind, we hate their gut for something they have done, but it all boils back to the fact that we are the ones affected by the grudges we hold. Humorously, I have seen people hold grudges for those they see on the internet. People enjoying themselves not knowing that you have a grudge against them. Grudges hurt you and not those you hold it again and if you want a chance to be happy, then avoid holding grudges for anyone.

Balance work and life

These are two different aspects of your life you want to avoid mixing up. If you do, one will suffer for the other, and when this happens, someday, somehow, you will see how much you have lost, not taking out time to balance both sides of your life. For instance, if you open a new business, every fiber in your being would be pushed to making sure that it succeeds, but it should not be at the expense of your family and life; you need to find a balance. If you do not, you will wake up one day to a distant wife, children you do not know, and a family who you barely are a part of. If you can find the balance, you would give room for every part of your life without letting one suffer for the other.

Help others and take care of yourself

Knowing that you are born for a purpose in life, you need to find ways to help those around you. Look for a way to give back to your community, and you would be glad you did. You should also make sure you take care of yourself and your health because only a healthy man can be wealthy.

Bottom Line

Happiness is a choice and a choice you must make if you want to enjoy your life. When life becomes difficult, happiness will help you pull through. When you hit roadblocks, happiness would help you pull through. When the going gets tough, only the happy would be the small shed of light at the corner because they are not too busy worrying about the bad side of things.

CHAPTER 8
Overcoming Obstacles

"Obstacles don't have to stop you. If you run into a wall, don't turn around and give up. Figure out how to climb it, go through it, or work around it."

Michael Jordan

For someone trying to become someone in life, someone different from who they have been, there are so many obstacles that would be faced. You can either break them down or let them limit your moving forward. These obstacles are stumbling blocks that hinder a person from reaching set goals. They are also known as limiting factors. You have to be determined to heal before you can take action. Once you have set your heart to heal, you will be able to overcome every obstacle that might rear its ugly head. Remember, setting goals is not what is important; actualizing and achieving them is what is of great importance. When executing these goals, life can become very unbearable. Unexpected setbacks would be on the path to success, just waiting in line to know the action you will take and mock you if they are given a chance to.

There is a saying that every success comes with its challenges. This is not entirely true because these challenges are roadmaps to success. They are problems that need to be solved to get to the next phase. It's just like *The Escape Room*. You have to solve one puzzle after another to be able to get out. This is how life is.

Are these obstacles significant to making life better? Are these obstacles necessary for dealing with the hard part of life?

Importance of Obstacles

There are much importance of obstacles, some of which are already known. Still, we would be looking at a few reasons why obstacles are essential for knowledge acquisition's sake. They are explained below;

- **Obstacles help you find purpose**: According to Angeline Trevena, some people see a wall and assume it is the end of their journey. Others see that same wall and decide that it is just the beginning. Purpose can be found when you stop focusing on your troubles. Instead, you should find ways to make yourself happy; find happiness. By lifting others, you can rise above any obstacle. You will be able to heal in the process.
- **Obstacles help you focus only on the things that count**: It is not everything that matters in this life. One has to focus on the goals one has set for themselves. They have to pursue their mission on Earth. You cannot do this if you do decide to heal. You have to have a clear mindset on the goals you intend to achieve. If you seek change, then change. If you

desire financial stability, go for it. If you want to be successful, what is stopping you from doing that? Large obstacles are formed by the accumulation of tiny obstacles. Suppose you think dodging one obstacle after another is the right choice. In that case, you might be making lots of mistakes, thereby accumulating more obstacles. Once you have a clear objective, overcoming obstacles would be a chicken change. While focusing on the things that count, ensure you have enough clues and directions to get by. Being uncertain would increase your limitations. The point I am trying to make is that you need to be very clear about the goals you wish to achieve. You need to focus on healing.

- **Obstacles show you who you really are**: Self-healing comes with identifying yourself. There are some challenges we would face that would rip your life apart. When this happens, you would be left with two choices. Do you want to know who you truly are, or would you prefer not to? It is not every time we are given the opportunity to realize our full potential, our full capabilities. When attempting to stretch yourself beyond your limits, you will definitely face obstacles. Once your limitations have been shown to you, you have to take the necessary steps to deal with them. You will be forced to overcome the barriers that will help define you; show you your true self.
- **Obstacles toughen you**: It is said that it is impossible for a person to be able to withstand challenges naturally. It is not a personal trait. It is a decision one has to make. Every living soul has obstacles to overcome. Why they are here is not to

make you desperate for help or ruin your peace of mind. They are here to toughen you up, to give you courage. Don't you think it is best to change your present circumstance to improve yourself?

- **Obstacles help lead the way**: There is a saying I came up with; you could climb the Mount. Everest; you only need to know where to place your feet. These obstacles, these stumbling blocks, can help create paths that would lead to the next phase of your life. For example, if you keep hurting yourself, your feelings, your emotions, the situation permits you to learn to forgive. There is always a solution to everything. All you need to do is shift your perspective. Let that action uncover teachable lessons. As Benjamin Franklin once said, the things which hurt, instruct.

In life, there are different types of obstacles. Every challenge a person faces can be grouped into three (3) separate categories;

- Internal obstacles,
- External or environmental obstacles,
- Habitual obstacles, and
- Social obstacles.

Internal obstacles are those obstacles that we can quickly solve by self-improvement. For instance, you can become financially stable by learning to save. You can get better at a job by improving your skill set. You can become a better you by making use of some personal development tips.

External or environmental obstacles are those obstacles we have little or no control over. They are seen as unexpected circumstances or occurrences. Because they are unforeseen, we are not fully prepared to deal with them. This is why we have to gather as much knowledge as possible to deal with them. Some of these obstacles include the economy and natural disasters – earthquakes, typhoons, whirlwinds, etc.

Personal or habitual obstacles are those obstacles that are of our doing. They are related to our behaviors, our psychology, as well as our mindset. These obstacles can only be gotten rid of by changing our habits. They prevent us from achieving our dreams; they stop us from moving forward. They also prevent us from making the right decisions that would help create a form of momentum which would take us to the finish line.

Social obstacles are related to people who do not wish for you to be a success. They are people who are ready to sabotage your efforts or are not prepared to take responsibility for their actions. These people would mess with your mind whenever you wish to take charge of situations. They would make you make the worst decisions. Every chance they get, they would try to manoeuvre your every word, every move.

To overcome any obstacles, the first thing you need to do is find out the category the obstacles you are facing fall into. Once that is done, you can then map out plans to solve them.

Before we find out ways to overcome your obstacles, there are some questions you need to ask yourself. This way, you will be able to take the proper steps to overcome these challenges.

Questions to be asked to Overcome Obstacles

- What are the things that indicate that you have a problem?
- How sure are you that these problems are yours to bear?
- How sure are you that they are accurate?
- Where did the problems you are sure you have originated from?
- What things perpetuated them?
- When did it happen?
- How did it happen?
- If you ignore these problems, what do you think would happen?
- Would the problem escalate or diminish?
- What would be the outcome?
- How does your problem affect other people?
- How does it affect your life?
- Would resolving those problems cause more problems or not?
- Do you control your behaviour?
- Do you control the behaviour of others?
- What part of the problem you are facing do you control?
- What aspect can you not control?
- How do you respond to the part you cannot control?
- What good thing is happening in your life?

- What thoughts, assumptions run through your mind?
- How do they contribute to the problem you are facing?
- What perspective is yet to be considered?
- Do you know anyone who has successfully overcome such a problem?
- What lessons have you learned from such a person?
- If you were to do anything differently, what would you do?
- Which of your family and friends would be of assistance?
- Have you attempted to find a solution(s)?
- How would you know your problem has been resolved?
- What criterion is needed for success?

As you take every step to achieve success, you will find answers to the questions listed above.

Steps to Overcome Obstacles

Rather than letting those obstacles get in your way, why not take the necessary steps to get rid of them?

STEP ONE: ANALYZE THE OBSTACLES

- **Find out what is holding you back**: How can we achieve this? Take a seat and think deeply. Find out the things that stand in your way of achieving your goals. Be as specific as possible. Know what your goals are and why it seems very hard for you to meet them. For you to map out a course of action, you will have to be aware of yourself. When mapping out a list, do not put your everyday complaint in it. It might mess up your list and your plan too. If you are having problems prioritizing your time, then your problem might be procrastination. If your problem is financial instability, it might be you lack motivation and understanding to make money.

- **Think about the origination of the obstacle**: One of the questions asked was, "Where did the problems you are sure you have originated from?" What thoughts, what habit keeps the obstacles strong? What are the things that prevent you from working through them? Once you have provided answers to these questions, you will be able to identify the changes to be made. For instance, you have adapted to a lifestyle of going to the gym three days a week; but after moving to a new environment with your family, you feel your movement is being restricted; you find it hard to keep up with the lifestyle. This would sap you of all motivation. What do you do in this case? The answer is simple; you look for alternatives.

- **Find obstacles that are similar to the ones you are facing**: Take some time to think of certain obstacles you have encountered at some point in your life and how you got rid of them. Figure out the approach you used; if it worked for you at that time or not. Learn from your past experience to enable you to work on the present obstacle.

- **Find out the things you can and cannot control**: There are some obstacles we face that might seem beyond our control. They sometimes seem so daunting because we are not looking at it from a positive angle. These obstacles are sometimes accompanied by negative emotions such as fear. How then can you determine the things you can control and the ones you cannot? Ask yourself what you can control, take a pen and paper and write down the actions you intend to take. Before we move on to the next tip, understand that you can control your behaviour, your attitude. You can control the effort you put into the things you do. You can also influence the decisions you make when an opportunity arises. You can control what you think about, what you eat, whatever action you take to move forward.

- **Analyses and break down interpersonal issues**: This is categorized under social obstacles. One of the many obstacles that can be frustrating is people. People are the main reason for a whole lot of problems we face in life. Negative emotions can cause us to make the wrong call. It can also make it impossible to work on our issues. What can we do about it? You must first break down your problems; then, find out what exactly stands in your way. There is a saying that it takes two to tango. In this case, it takes two to create an obstacle and contribute to it. Develop mental stoppers. Mental stoppers are behaviors, words, actions that can help control your anger and think rationally. One common mental stopper is counting from one to ten. While analysing interpersonal issues, try listening to the problems of others and think of them from their own perspective. Solving the problems of others may proffer solutions to your problem too. Better still, you can restructure your interaction with other people to avoid more issues.

STEP TWO: CHANGE YOUR PERCEPTIONS

- **Recognize it as a phase:** True, you have obstacles in front of you, and you have to face them. How do you cope? How do you deal with them? You must understand the world changes; time changes; everything changes. Change, they say, is constant. The only thing that can never change is the sun rising in the East and setting in the West. The obstacles you are facing right now are not forever. Always remind yourself that the challenges you face will soon pass.
- **Remind yourself of the good things in your life:** Life comes with its good and bad days. Most people find it very hard to see the good things in their life because the bad ones have clouded everything. Because of this, they find it hard to remember the good things of life. Spend as much time as you can to enjoy the things of life.
- **Stay flexible:** To change your perception, you must stay as flexible as possible always. You might decide to go against the flow, which might not be a good thing, but you might end up slapping into very high walls (obstacles). But if you decide to go with the flow, any direction the wind takes you, go with it.
- **Stay challenged and be grateful for them:** When you keep taking the easy path of life, being challenged would be difficult. Do not run away from them; let them happen. Take risks when you can. You'll never know the promises they carry. It is just like trying to start up a business. First, you would need to source for capital, business site, advertise to

get customers and retain them, ensure there is a steady stream of products and income, etc. These are obstacles that are to be overcome. It might take a while to accomplish them but take it one step at a time, alright?

- **Believe in yourself:** While facing obstacles, you must be ready to overcome them, and to do so, you must learn to believe in yourself. Self-confidence and self-esteem are crucial in this case. Doubting yourself would bring about indecisiveness and take away everything good from your experiences in life. Which life experience would you prefer, the positive or the negative experiences?

STEP THREE: OVERCOME THE OBSTACLES

- **Break your problems into smaller bits**: As mentioned before, you can break your major issues into smaller ones and work on them bit by bit. No one can travel around the world in one day, or should I use the famous saying, Rome was not built in a day. It was built one grain of sand after another. Break the mountain of problems you have into smaller chunks. Write them down, and then ask yourself what obstacles prevent you from solving the issues listed one after the other. For instance, if your goal is to heal yourself, one looming obstacle would be accepting your weaknesses. Once this is taken care of, the rest would come easy.
- **Find a more creative solution to your problems**: After listing your problems, the next thing to do is find more than one solution. You might ask, "Is it possible to reach my goal while trying to avoid those obstacles entirely? There might

be some shortcuts that one can take, but they do not always work. While attempting to take those shortcuts, you can talk to someone who has already gotten past similar obstacles. Such a person might be very familiar with the routes you are taking or intend to take. They might even be familiar with routes you have not heard of.

- **Have an action plan in place**: Putting your goals on paper is so you will not forget them. Just writing them is not the only thing to do. You have to put them in prominent places. When jotting down your plans, you must first begin with the present day and end it with achieving the goal for the day. As you learn, you tend to grow and face more obstacles than you expect. In the process, you can adapt your plan to find the best path.

- **Monitor your progress**: Keeping track of your progress while working towards the accomplishment of your goal. It would not hurt to keep a journal, writing down your achievements as well as your setbacks. Set milestones, and do not forget to reward yourself after every achievement made.

- **Advice and support are necessary**: It is not every advice a person gives to you that you should take. Sometimes, these advices are not for your own good but to favor the other. Another thing you should look out for is advice from biased individuals. You should be able to detect when an advice is given with all honesty and when it is not. Look for people who share goals similar to yours. Surround yourself with friends that will encourage you. Be accountable. Share your milestones with them. Share ideas and seek advice from those who are more experienced. You never know who might have overcome the same obstacles you are facing. Some so many people share the same habit, hobby, career, and emotional struggle. Look out for them.

- **Rid yourself of bad habits**: Bad habits are habits that are detrimental to the well being of a person. These habits may not seem like obstacles, but they can be setbacks. Treat them like obstacles; overcome them. Get rid of those setbacks.
- **Imagine your goals for motivation**: Motivations serve as encouragements. Close your eyes and picture yourself after overcoming the obstacles one at a time. Use such motivation to remind yourself why you are putting in a lot of effort and making sacrifices. Once you have gotten wind of all your obstacles, you will feel good. It does not mean you are free from every obstruction. Trust me, more will come, and when they do, you have to be ready.
- **Develop problem-solving skills**: If you already have problem-solving skills, hone them. Sometimes, decisions are made based on gut instincts. If you choose to make them, ensure you take an analytic approach - an approach you can use are worst-case scenarios. If you try doing something and do not succeed at all, what do you do? Will you give up or come up with a backup plan?

Understand that we were brought into this world for different reasons. We have the ability to do anything and become ourselves.

Getting rid of doubts, insecurities, low self-esteem and other negative behaviors and attributes are giant steps to healing. Though we all struggle to make our lives meaningful, we should always stay positive.

With the right skill sets, you can overcome your obstacles and grow from there. Without these skills, you might eventually be overwhelmed by these challenges. There are some other ways to overcome obstacles. They include:

- Using the power of motivation

- Winning the influence

Using the Power of Motivation

Motivation is very powerful and works for everyone. When an obstacle is set before you, motivation can give you the drive and the power to overcome whatever it is that comes your way. Here are some of the best ways to use motivation to overcome your obstacles:

Think outside the box

One of the most motivating ways to overcome obstacles is thinking outside the box. I remember the movie tower heist where they had to take a car through the elevator. It could not fit, so they put it on the elevator shaft and got it out the floor before the last; problem solved. They never thought inside the box but outside the box.

Remain motivated

Everything would happen at the right time; you just need to remain motivated to the point when it happens. Even though your plan does not materialize at the time, you would have loved it too; it would eventually happen. You just have to be patient enough for it to happen and remain motivated.

Review yourself

Everyone needs a check at some point, including you, and if you have not, you need to do it at once. For example, suppose there is something that prevents you from overcoming your obstacles like fear, guilt, and even low self-esteem. Be honest about it and think of the changes you need to make to overcome your obstacles. Sometimes, we are the ones holding ourselves back and not the obstacles, and until you overcome these mindsets, your obstacles would always be there.

Support Others

When push comes to shove, you need to make sure you support others and inspire them to overcome your obstacles. When you support others, you have many people who look up to you, sort of like a team that would help you overcome your obstacles without any stress.

Surrender Yourself

You do not have to control everything; sometimes, all you can do is leave the rest to fate. You just get to notice that some obstacles would eventually evaporate on their own, so it does not have to take over your life and existence.

With the right level of motivation, there is nothing you cannot overcome. You can achieve anything you set your mind to achieve with the right level of motivation because you are a winner.

Winning the Influence

Another thing you need to do is win the influence of others. You cannot do anything on your own, so you have to win the influence of others. You have to win the influence of those around you, building a team of people you trust to help you push barriers that are overly bigger than you. Here are some of the ways to win the influence of people:

Avoid criticizing or Condemning People

There are better ways to win people over than to condemn them. For example, when you compliment people and then look for a good way to point out their faults to them, they would be drawn to you, especially because you made them better without bringing them.

Praise People

Look for the good side of people and tell it to them. People who can see the good in people are scarce, and if you can be one of them, you can win the influence of others and overcome obstacles.

Call them by their name

If you cannot remember their names, they would feel like they are of no use to you. But if you can remember to call people by their names, it shows genuine interest in them.

Acknowledge it when you make mistakes

The best set of people are those who acknowledge their mistakes. If people who look up to you can see you acknowledge your mistakes, you can influence them, and together you can overcome obstacles.

You have the power to win, and you can win when you overcome the obstacles on your way, as we have highlighted in this chapter of this book.

CHAPTER 9
How to Heal Yourself

Just to give you a heads-up, we would be having a lot of quotes from Louise L. Hay, author of the best-seller, "You Can Change Your Life". Our first quote, coming right up ...

"In the infinity of life where I am, all is perfect, whole and complete.

I believe in a power far greater than I am that flows through me, every moment of every day.

I open myself to the wisdom within, knowing that there is only One Intelligence in this Universe.

Out of this One Intelligence come all the answers, all the solutions, all the healings, all the new creations.

I trust this Power and Intelligence, knowing that whatever I need to know is revealed to me and that whatever I need comes to me in the right time, space and sequence.

All is well in my world."

I believe in the saying that life is not as complicated as we see it. It is actually quite simple. What we give to life is what it gives back in return. Our thoughts become our truths. We are responsible for whatever action we take. It does not matter if it is the best or the worst action. Through our thoughts, we create our experiences. Through our feelings, our actions are created too. We make our experiences, our situations and lose power over them. We begin to blame others for our shortcomings that we forget it was our doing. Do not let anyone or anything have power over you. We can easily create balance in our minds. Every individual believes that different experiences can be made; correct me if I am wrong. This belief then becomes true to us.

Our thoughts and beliefs are backed by the Universe. It is no wonder that we are always told to think positive thoughts, as negativity would easily be attached to our lives. No matter the problem we are facing, the outer effects of our inner thoughts are our experiences. Hating ourselves is hating the way we think of ourselves. It seems like everyone on Earth is suffering from self-guilt of different degrees, which should not be the case. There are ways in which a person can heal. Still, before we do, we have to understand that every illness from the different aspects of life comes from a state of unforgiveness. We must learn to forgive. Forgiveness gives room to a healthy life. You must learn to get go of every "stressful" object, behaviour, and individual. Forgiveness is not just about saying, "I forgive you"; it is about being willing to do so. How to forgive is up to the Universe to work on. Love yourself, and approve of yourself.

Quoting Louise;

"In the infinity of life where I am, all is perfect, whole and complete.

I am always divinely protected and guided.

It is safe for me to look within myself.

It is safe for me to look into the past.

It is safe for me to enlarge my viewpoint of life.

I am far more than my personality; past, present, or future.

I now choose to rise above my personality problems, to recognize the magnificence of my being.

I am totally willing to learn to love myself.

All is well in my world."

I try as much as I can to repeat this quote every day and make it a part of me. I advise you do the same. It can change your negative thought life and give you peace of mind. To heal, you must first decide to change. Decide to be willing to change. Once the decision has been made, begin to do some mental work. Examine your thoughts; examine your belief. Notice the repairs and replacements to be made.

The ways in which one can heal includes the following;

- **Awareness**: This is the first step to self-healing. Some patterns are buried within us. You just have to be aware of them if you want to be healed. While attempting to be aware, we might think it is a silly thing to do, but it is not. It might seem unacceptable to your mode of thinking. You might be thinking, "I don't think I can do it; I don't want to do it." Because of this, your resistance comes up strong. The thought of doing it might cause you to become angry. Another form of resistance that might come up is impatience. Impatience becomes a resistance to change. You need to acknowledge your responsibility; recognize the power within you. Let it transform your thoughts into personal experiences. What is the hardest thing you intend to accomplish? Do you resist it much? If so, then you are looking at the greatest lesson yet to be learned. You need to give up that resistance. Allow yourself to understand what you should. Once that is accomplished, the next step to take would come easy. Do not, by any chance, let your resistance stop you from making the correct change. Specific actions show our resistance. They are categorized under the following;
- Assumptions
- Beliefs
- Denial
- Fear
- Nonverbal cues

- Self-conception

ASSUMPTIONS:

These are conclusions that are made based on little or no facts. These assumptions are made to justify your resistance. Some of the statements we come up with are;

- You would not understand.

- Our cases are entirely different.

- Trust me, only crazy people visit therapists.

- No one can help with my problem.

- No good will come out of it anyway.

BELIEFS:

While growing up, we were made to believe some things, and those things have been a hindrance to our becoming someone in life. Some of these beliefs include;

- It is not right.

- It is not done.

- Spiritual people would not take such action.

- My parents did not do such, so I won't.

- It is pretty expensive.

- It will take forever.

- I am not that kind of person.

DENIAL

This form of resistance creeps in when you try to deny the need to change. We make sentences like;

- It is fine.
- I was alright the last time.
- What difference would the change make?
- I would rather ignore it, with the hope that the problem would go away.

FEAR

This is one of the most significant categories of resistance. Most people are not scared of everything but the fear of the unknown. The statements they make include;

- I will fail.
- It might be expensive.
- I am not ready.
- I am afraid to voice out.
- It is hard for me to accomplish.
- I just can't do it.
- I would rather die.

- I may lose my freedom in the process.

- It might ruin my life.

- I am not perfect.

- I lack the strength.

- I do not want anyone to know I have problems.

- I don't want to be mocked.

- I do not want to talk about it.

The list is endless. Let us look for some resistance in the examples below:

Example I:

A friend of mine came to me and said she was in a lot of emotional pain. Her family was in jeopardy. Her younger brother had an accident, her mother had a stroke because she was overthinking. Her father was deceased (God rest his soul), and she was not making enough money to cater to the needs of the rest of the family. She felt comfortable telling me her problems, but when I began to talk, to try to advise her, she began to feel uncomfortable. My guess was, she has heard these before but has not done anything about it because she fears the unseen. When I give a piece of advice, she brings up an excuse. She was building walls around her. I felt she was not ready to be healed. She was not prepared to get rid of all her barriers, her resistance.

Example II: There was a friend of mine who had lumps in her breasts for eleven years. When she first noticed it, she didn't see it as anything. She thought it was just tissue that would dissolve in no time. As the months rolled by, she self-monitored the lumps to be sure they were not growing. They were two in number at the time but later became three. As the years rolled by, the fear that it might become malignant increased. She was afraid of going to the hospital. After much encouragement, she started visiting the hospital. Every year, she goes for check-ups. She was always told it is benign, but you have to get rid of it. This made matters worse for her because it increased her fear. As the lumps kept growing, her fear kept growing. I begged her to have it removed. She started coming up with so many excuses that I could count. Some of them were, "What if they make a mistake?", "What if all the tests were wrong?", "What if they remove more than is necessary?", "What if they conclude that my breasts have to be removed?" To be honest, I tried answering all her questions, but she did not believe any of them. She was not ready to do something about her predicament.

What were their resistances? What is your resistance?

LET YOUR FRIENDS BE

Sometimes, we forget that we can take care of ourselves and expect people to take care of us. We forget that we can make that change we so desire without the help of others. But sadly, rather than working on our transition, we pay attention to the change that our friends need. The fact that we do not focus on the change we need simply shows that we are resisting. The lack of focus is the resistance. When something works according to plan, we tend to share it with others, but we keep them to ourselves when they do not. The truth is, we may not be ready to change how we see our problems or learn to find solutions to them. It is pretty hard to make those changes. If your friends are resistant to changing your life; to healing, leave them alone. Work on yourself.

TAKE A LOOK AT YOURSELF

There is a practice I tell people who find themselves in this situation to practice. It is called Mirror Work. The function of a mirror is to show you what you look like, inversely. But in this case, the mirror would be reflecting how we feel about ourselves. It will clearly show us the areas we need to change to heal, to live a peaceful life. Why not look into the eyes of your reflection. Every time you pass a mirror, say something positive about yourself. As far as I am concerned, this is the best way to make affirmations. Look into a mirror and proclaim positivity into your life. Say it out loud. While taking this action, you will become fully aware of the resistance you have set up, and it would be easier for you to move through it. How do you feel? What negative beliefs are you holding on to? What thoughts are still limbering in your mind? Despite thinking about these things, you should not scold yourself. It is not the right time to do it. What you should be doing is paying attention to the things that are going on and the beliefs that are rising up to the surface. The feelings and beliefs that are rising up to the surface are the ones that are problematic to you. Can you recognize where they originated from? While affirming and you feel nothing, it is not that your affirmations are not working. It simply means that you have to try something else before you begin to affirm.

SEE YOUR NEEDS THROUGH REPEATED PATTERNS

For every attitude, every habit you have, every experience you are going through, there is a pattern. For every pattern repeated, there is a need for them. The needs tend to correspond with some of the feelings and beliefs you have. There is something deep within us that needs the problems we have, the problems we face. How many times have you made statements like, "I will never do it again" or "I will not be a part of it anymore"? But before the day or the weekends, you find yourself doing the same thing. If you see yourself doing the same thing repeatedly, it means that you do not have discipline. You lack the willpower to change. Because you are weak, you might just end up adding more guilt to the one you already have.

BE WILLING TO RELEASE THE NEED

For whatever condition you are in, there is a need in you for it. Take a step back and work on that need. Be ever-willing to release it. Once you have gotten rid of that need, you will not have the desire to perform such an action again. Affirm that you are ready and willing to release the need to create resistance. If you keep resisting the will and the need to heal, your affirmations would be for nothing. The walls we build around ourselves need to be broken down.

DO NOT PROCRASTINATE

Procrastination is created by self-doubt. Procrastination is a way of keeping things from happening at the right time. It is a way of stopping yourself from being where you ought to be. Those who procrastinate spend more time and energy reducing their self-esteem and blaming themselves. They see themselves as lazy and tag themselves like that. These negative affirmations make them see themselves as bad people. Procrastination stops a person from moving forward. They hinder people from becoming who they want to be, from achieving what they ought to accomplish at the given time.

DO NOT RESENT THE GOOD OF OTHERS

I know someone who was an attention-seeker. He did not do good things to get attention. He did unspeakable things just to be noticed. I remember a time when he assaulted our class teacher just to be seen. He was sent to the principal's office more times than I can count. He became known as the school tyrant. His name was Ben. Ben would come late to class just because. He would fail to do the class assignment because he wanted to be called out in class. His reason for doing what he did was because he longed to have something to call his own. He saw other people get noticed because they do good things, but whenever he does good, he does not get noticed. When he sees someone getting recognized for the good they do, rather than rejoice with them, he resents them. The resentment he felt became a barrier to his change, to his healing. Do not resent the good of others. It would do you no good.

DO NOT CRITICIZE YOURSELF

Self-criticism has to do with scolding yourself for things done. I know someone who is overweight and has been striving to become fit. But whenever she tries working out and gets no positive result, she becomes angry with herself and ends up stress-eating. Within an hour, she would have finished eating the big bowl of ice cream in the freezer. She would order two boxes of pizza and eat whatever food she finds. Then she sleeps. The next day, she wakes up and begins to hate herself for overeating and adding to the problem she already has. When she was growing up, eating a big bowl of ice cream was not seen as a bad thing because her parents always laughed and thought it cute. She also lived in a house that made eating seem very important. They made eating very important. When it's breakfast time, the table is always filled with more than one can eat, and everyone is expected to eat to their fill. It seemed like the family approved of eating a lot. Because of that, whenever she tries to do something and does not achieve what she had in mind, she goes back to eating a bowl of ice cream. When you scold yourself, who do you think you would blame? Who do you think you are treating poorly? You are only hurting yourself, and that is like adding more fuel to the fire. Bear in mind that what was done in the past is the past. Make your present and future work for you. Be very kind to yourself; learn to love yourself. Approve of your actions. Stay positive!

Louise provided us with a beautiful quote. It is advised that you say it every morning when you wake up.

"In the infinity of life where I am, all is perfect, whole and complete.

I see any resistance patterns within me only as something else to release.

They have no power over me.

I am the power in my world.

I flow with the changes taking place in my life as best as I can.

I approve of myself and the changes happening within me.

I am doing the best I can.

Each day gets easier.

I rejoice that I am in the rhythm and flow of my ever-changing life.

Today is a beautiful day.

I choose to make it so.

All is well in my world."

UNDERGO THE PROCESS OF LOVING YOURSELF

It does not matter the problem you are facing; you must work on trying to love yourself. Loving yourself is a solution to most, if not all your problems. Remember the times you felt good about yourself. When you love yourself, you feel good about yourself. Making reference to the example used before, "the ice-cream-eating girl," she was trying to be fit at the beginning, right? This means she had little love for her physical body. But the love was not enough because whenever she looks at herself and sees no result, she goes back to her old habit. Loving yourself would require patience, determination, care, approval, and acceptance of self. Did she approve of herself? Did she accept herself? Loving yourself would help rid your mind of criticism. You might begin to ask yourself questions like, "How can I possibly like myself?", "What can I possibly like about myself?" or "If I do not criticize myself, how will I change?" To love yourself, specific processes must be followed. They are explained below;

- **Train your mind**: As we already know, self-criticism is something of the mind. It is when the mind tries to analyse some things you have done and passes judgment. It makes you wish you did not do it that way. Your mind points out your faults and shortcomings. To train your mind, you will have to practice the mirror work. Make positive affirmations to your reflection. Once that is done, learn to forgive yourself. How do you feel after this exercise? For positive changes, you will have to learn to accept and approve of yourself. It is one of the many ways you can heal. Making positive affirmations is a guarantee that brings up everything buried in your consciousness. When negative thoughts come up, remember to think positive ones. Let the positive ones overshadow the negative ones.

- **Practice awareness**: While training your mind, think happy thoughts. Do things that make you feel alive; that make you feel good about yourself. Be surrounded by people who make you feel good about yourself, not the ones who keep criticizing you all the time.

- **Reinforce new learning**: There are lots of ways a person can reinforce the things they learn. Some of these ways include; putting affirmations on paper, meditating, exercising, eating good food, performing mental exercises like visualization and reading.

- **Have no belief in limitations**: There is a saying that the sky is the limit. I disagree. I believe the sky is just the starting point, and there is no limit. When faced with trying situations, do not let negative thoughts get in the way. While believing there are no limitations, do not forget to love yourself. Imagine being the person you are working towards, expanding your knowledge, awareness, and understanding of how the mind works.

While practicing all these, do not forget to demonstrate the results. Do whatever you can to ensure to experience a positive transformation, a change in your life that would bring you joy and pleasure.

"There is something beautiful about all scars of whatever nature. A scar means the hurt is over; the wound is closed and healed, done with."
Harry Crews

"The inevitable part of life is pain. However, the choice to suffer is yours."
Pain Paseda Oluwafemi

As we have highlighted in this quote, we would all face pains and disappointments at some point in time or the other, but the choice to suffer is up to you. To move on in life, you need to be able to self-heal. You need to put yourself together and recover from whatever it is you are experiencing, and this chapter has just the thing for you. Here are some other ways to heal yourself from any situation and circumstance.

Never think of giving up

The minute you have the thought of throwing in the towel, you have given the challenge the upper hand. You need to understand that this is a fight you can win; therefore, you need to avoid the thought of giving up. If you do not allow this thought to grow, you will end up winning. If you do not allow the thought of giving up to become an option, then you would overcome and eventually heal.

Heal your soul by reducing stress

Stress has been made part and parcel of who we are, but for someone who wants to heal, you need to let go of the handle. You need to give yourself some time off to heal because you cannot heal from deep within if you do not. So, you take some time off from work and everything, stressing you to cool down and let your body recover. When you do this, your body focuses on the single task at hand, which is total recovery from the thing you are trying to recover from and nothing else. Not work, not getting to an appointment, nothing but recovery.

Love yourself

This is an important part of healing, and you must realize it. Nobody can love you as much as you love yourself. So, if you do not love "you," then you rely on the love of others for comfort. So, if you lost something or someone you loved as a result of overlooking yourself and making them the center of your existence, then you need to start loving yourself more.

When you prioritize loving yourself, you would not be pained when people do not act accordingly. When you love yourself, nobody can bring you down. If things do not work out with a job, a relationship, or anything, you just make yourself understand that that job or person is not worth you being down. Of course, some situations are tougher than others, but you can recover from anything when you love yourself.

Boost your energy

Boosting your energy is a call to avoid all the things that bring you down. Anything that brings you down should be avoided by all means, leaving you to choose only positive vibes and things that bring you emotional comfort and not the other way around. When you embrace positive energy around you, you have a boost of energy, which helps you heal yourself from practically anything.

Try the things you enjoy

We all have something that we enjoy, something that makes us happy. These are things you should embrace on your journey towards healing from anything. Avoid stressors and working too hard else, you would find that your life gets overly complicated than it ought to be. On your road to healing, anything that makes you smile is an option – well, anything good.

Reset your life

Sometimes, you just have to hit the reset button on your road to healing. You need to go back to the drawing table and see if you are in the best place. For example, you might be trying to heal, and the only thing holding you back would be your environment. If you find yourself in this position, you need to make sure you take time to reset and see what stops you from healing.

Bottom Line

Everyone has the chance and capacity to heal from anything. You just need to be ready to embrace your situation. Then, if you can, you would recover, become a better person, and even stronger because you have overcome what would make most people give up.

CHAPTER 10
Rules of Living A Good Life

Are you happy? How do you feel about the life you have today? Do you think you are living your best life? Is your daily life filled with excitement or doubts? Do you feel contented with your life at the moment? If your answers are negative, it means you are not living a good life. It also means that you are not following the correct rules of living a good life. I have heard people say, I do not know what my life would bring tomorrow, so I just live it as it comes. They do not plan their days. They have no idea what to do to make their lives better. Everyone must be able to live their lives to the fullest. Remember, the experiences of your life are yours to create. We all indeed have good and bad days, but letting the bad days get to you is something that must not happen. What is essential is to make the best of all your days. Remember, unlike cats, we have only one life to live. There is no way we can control everything that occurs on a daily. You can only control how you behave towards them. This way, you will be able to shape your future as you want it and live well.

Quoting Steve Jobs, "Your time on Earth is limited. Do not waste it living the life of another person. Do not be trapped by dogma, which is living the result of what other people think. Do not let the noise of the opinion of others drown your inner voice. Most importantly, be courageous enough to follow your heart and your intuition. Both of them know what you really want to become. See every other thing as secondary."

There are so many rules to be followed to live a good life. It is high time we get your good life going. We would be taking a look at some rules of living a good life.

30 Rules of Living a Good Life

1. Begin your day on a clean slate: Do not let the mistake of yesterday ruin our today. I have made this mistake one too many times. Sometimes, when I fail to accomplish something the day before, I think about the things I should have to make it work until I fall asleep. When I wake up, it is the first thing I remember. I am not saying you should not work on your previous mistake. What I am telling you to do is not allow it to ruin your day. Do not let it hold you back. Remember, life is short, so make every moment count.

2. Be true to yourself: This is quite difficult for people who desire to place others rather than themselves. A people-pleaser would find it very difficult to live for themselves. These people have no idea what path their life is supposed to take, and they rely on people to show them the way. It is

crucial that you maintain the original version of yourself and not become a duplicate of another.

3. Stay committed to your growth and development: While trying to heal, try to self-reflect. Use the opportunity to build your strength. Relying on feelings of familiarity might do you no good. Instead, pay more attention to the things that would help you grow more.

4. Learn to think of the future: Most people think, "what if I did this, what if I did that." They forget that there is always a 'next time.' Rather than focusing on things they can work on; they focus on what they should have done. So, concentrating on things you can work on is the best thing to do in any situation you find yourself in.

5. Let your life be aligned with purpose: Have you found out the reason why you are alive? Do you have an idea of the purpose you are to fulfil? If no, then there is still some work you have to do. If yes, congratulations! But the real question is, are you letting your life be aligned with the purpose you have already found? What are the things you can do to let your life be totally aligned with your purpose? Can you be true to your purpose always? Answer these questions, and you would be taking a step to living a good life.

6. Create a personal manual: Create a personal handbook for yourself. Let it be a manual to live a good life. Like every manual, your personal manual should contain your mission

statement, vision, values, strengths, and weaknesses, as well as action plans.

7. Set ideal goals: Before goals can be fixed, one has to decide the kind of life they want to live. They have to design it themselves. Ask yourself if you want to fully be in charge of your life or not. Know what you want out of the life you intend to live. Once that is done, you can set long-term and short-term goals, or as you see fit. Be specific on the goals you plan to achieve. The more detailed your goals are, the better.

8. Indulge in the things you love: As mentioned before, life is too short. It is also very precious. It is so precious that one should not be denied of the things that they enjoy. If you do not enjoy something, do not waste time doing them. You might achieve something beneficial from it or not. Use your time and energy to do things that would bring you joy, happiness, and fulfilment.

9. Believe in yourself: To do this, you must first develop a belief system. A belief system is something that gives your life meaning and how the world is seen. Be comfortable with the system of belief you have developed. Your belief system should be your belief. In this case, your belief system should be "believing in yourself." You do not have to prove anything to anyone but yourself. You do not justify your actions. While developing a belief system, you have to be aware of your limitations. It is the first step to making your dreams

come true. You must first realize that you are a human being. This means you will have certain strengths and weaknesses. It also means that you would be prone to mistakes, but rather than feeling bad about yourself, use the errors to your advantage. Remember, no one is perfect. Even with all you wish to accomplish, you need to understand that you are still human. You are not perfect, and you need to understand that. So, you need to believe you can go far in life and accomplish all you want to, but you need to also know your limits. You need to set goals but goals that are realistic. Imagine a skinny guy setting a goal to be the heavyweight champion of the UFC. It is not only unrealistic; it puts unnecessary pressure on the individual. So, cut yourself some slack set goals you can enjoy as you ride through the tides of life.

10. Be unique: We are unique in different ways. Comparing yourself with other people makes you less unique. I remember when I was much younger, I felt I was not successful enough. I was constantly comparing my success with that of my friends; I thought they were doing everything right. Whenever I made a mistake, I was always embarrassed to admit it. Later on, I later realized that it was only robbing me of my happiness. I was able to maintain my uniqueness and peace of mind by unleashing my true greatness. This was achieved by doing what I love, not comparing myself with others, and love everyone as I loved myself. We are made differently. We are given different

paths to walk. As diverse as we are, different gifts, talents, and opportunities are bestowed upon us. Have it in mind that we are all embarking on the journey to find our truths. Without happiness, everything we do is meaningless.

11. Let forgiveness come easy to you: Is it possible to forgive everyone for anything they do to you? The answer is yes. It does not matter how hurt you are. When you forgive people, you tend to have this inner peace. Inner peace is the greatest treasure anyone can have. There is a saying that forgiveness is the medicine of the soul. So, to heal, you must learn to forgive yourself and others too. Rid yourself of every negative emotion. Embrace lessons learned from everything that has occurred in your life. With hope, focus on the future.

12. Fix your problems or deal with them: One lesson I have learned about life is that people who complain a lot are often neglected by others. No one likes people who complain a lot. Trust me, everyone has their own problems and is trying to deal with them. No one wants to be a bearer of the problem of others. Do not blame others for your problems. Do not make excuses for yourself. Work on that problem that is giving you a headache. Do not be a drama queen. It does not help. Rather than complain, find a solution. You can talk to people about your problem, not because you want to pour everything on them, but because you need help finding a solution to those problems.

13. Have a plan: Having a plan involves creating a map, a route, a target, a strategy for your life. Having a plan tells you that you have a place to go, you have something to achieve. Having a plan also indicates that you have thought about your life, and like most people, you are willing to go through life one step at a time. Work out the things you intend to do, take the proper steps to achieve the goals, and move forward. When making plans understand that it is not a dream. It is something you intend to do. Another thing you must understand is that when you make a plan, it does not mean you will have to follow it to the latter. There are times when you have to make adjustments. For example, when going according to the plans you have fixed, you might meet certain obstacles on the way. When you do, you have to make changes. Do not set rigid goals because of the changes that can occur. If you do not plan your plan well, you will keep dreaming.

14. Be well-mannered: If I ask you if you have good manners, I am sure your answer would be yes. Everyone believes they have good manners. But when you are under stress, you would notice your manners would begin to slip. If you are honest with yourself, you would admit that you tend to act irrationally towards others whenever there is a shake in your life. In this situation, you should not forget to follow the rules. Some of the behaviors that tell if you are well-mannered or not, do the following;

15. Try complimenting people when it is needed. If they do not deserve the compliments, do not go throwing the compliments around.

16. Do not put yourself in places you are not needed.

17. Learn to fulfil promises when made.

18. When people get in your way, learn to control your temper.

19. When you get into someone else's way, learn to apologize.

20. Learn to be hospitable when necessary.

21. Learn to be charming and courteous as often as you can.

22. Do not procrastinate: Procrastination is something a lot of people have trouble overcoming. What does procrastination mean? It simply means putting things that are to be done at a particular time on hold. It is a waste of time in your life. To overcome procrastination, you just have to do things when you are expected to. Do not hold it off till you feel it is the right time because there would be no right time.

23. Step out of your comfort zone: We all have our comfort zones, and we sometimes get too attached to them. When we grow too attached to our comfort zone, we are unable to learn new things. When you step out of your comfort zone, you will keep learning and growing.

24. Learn to think for yourself: You might think this rule is unnecessary considering that it is something everyone does

daily. What I mean by this rule is that you should be able to have a sense of identity and uphold it. It also means you should be very clear about your opinions. We are all vulnerable within us, but we do not show it because outward, we try to blend in. we all want to be loved and respected by others. We are sometimes tempted to wish to be whatever other people want us to be. This is where your originality comes into play. You have to be you. Be different. Being different does not mean you should see people as trash. Besides, if you treat people like dirt, you will be shunned. So, stay humble, kind, and you will be loved and accepted by all. Being all these does not mean you should be a feet-kisser. Stand up to yourself, your opinions, and be heard. To think yourself, you have to have something to think about and then do the thinking.

25. Do things that take you out of yourself: This is quite similar to leaving your comfort zone. Everyone has something positively different that pushes them in the right way. We all need that one thing that would take us out of ourselves for a bit. These things are to help us not to take ourselves too seriously. For example, for me, music helps bring me out of myself for a bit. It reminds me of the simple pleasures of life. It also gives me peace of mind. What thing takes you out of yourself?

26. Be the best in what you do: Most people find it hard to put their best and be the best in the things they do. They tend to

settle for less. If you intend to spend time doing the things you love, you might as well put your best into it. Do not settle for people who make you uncomfortable. Do not work with people who do not like what you do or do not expect you to have a say in anything. Do not settle for jobs you do not like. Also, do not pretend to be happy about things you are not comfortable with. Go for what you want and not what other people want you to.

27. Have a mentor: It is said that there is no better or faster way to accomplish your desired goals if you do not have a mentor or a role model. Their role in your life is to drive you to achieve more and share advice when it is needed. Your role models should serve as a reminder of what you intend to be and should push you to attain that expected goal.

28. Focus on the big picture: When setting goals, it is crucial to focus on small pictures, but it is imperative to focus on the bigger picture. With your eyes on the prize, you will be motivated to take the necessary steps to achieve it. Focusing on the bigger picture can help you get a lot from life.

29. Relish little moments: Every moment of your day should be considered precious. Your waking up every day should be appreciated. Be thankful that you are given the opportunity to see another day. Being kissed by the sun is another exciting thing. You might see it as nothing, but there are people who wish the sun could touch their skin. I know of a girl with a very rare condition. She cannot have her bath,

sweat, or let water touch her skin, else it would seem like she is dying. Her skin would react, she would be in severe pain and more. Remembering this makes me very grateful for being whole. Being with other people, going for walks in the park watching the sunset are wonderful things that should be cherished. These are the things that make up your life.

30. Understand that only you can change yourself: Do not expect people to behave the way you want them. Do not expect people around you to change because you want them to. Focus on the change you are to make yourself. This way, you would be able to know what you want when you want it and how you want it. This way, your life would be filled with joy and happiness. You would have the peace of mind you have always been craving.

31. See disappointments as stepping stones to success: Most people try to avoid disappointments. I, for one, have tried avoiding disappointments. I remember when I was planning to set up a business but did not have enough capital. I asked myself. "If I ask my friends, there is a probability that I would not get the answer I hope for." Before I even asked for the capital, I was already giving myself excuses. Because of that, I had to put a pause on the business I was planning to set up. Now the funny thing was after I put a halt to my business plan, I then shared my idea with my friends. Interestingly enough, they agreed to help me with capital. What I am trying to make you understand is that you should

not run away from disappointments. They are a part of what makes us human. Disappointments are a reflection of our real emotions. Rather than resisting it, simply embrace it.

32. Face your fears: Our fears make us human. We tend to fear everything. Our fear of the unknown, fear of risks, fear of facing the crowd, and every fear we can think of can prevent us from growing. So, rather than avoiding them, we should recognize them as stepping stones for growth. Face your fears, address them and overcome them.

33. Maximize your all: For one to live their best life, you must be able to maximize your soul, body, and mind. You need to make use of your being physically, spiritually, emotionally, and mentally. You might have all the money in the world but be having physical health issues. Do you think you are living a good life? What if you are in excellent health but have a poor mental state of mind? Do you call it living a good life? As long as one part of your life is faulty, you are not living a good life. Everything has to be balanced. Reserve no part of your life. Use every part of it.

34. Request for feedback when necessary: In life, human beings have blind spots. Some of these blind spots are visible to us; others are not. There are some blind spots that we have that are difficult to be identified. Because of this, it would not hurt to ask people for feedback. Why are feedbacks important? Feedbacks are vital because they provide you

with an additional perspective of yourself. When generating feedback from people, ensure the people are not biased.

35. Learn to advise yourself: In every human, there is a fountain of wisdom. The fountain of wisdom is what we call intuition. Making use of our intuition is not a rapid process but a gradual one. How can you make use of your intuition? The first step is to recognize the feeling or the small voice within you. That voice scolds you when you have done things you ought not to have done. You can refer to that voice as your conscience. It tells you when to do certain things. It tells you when to apologize, when to say thank you, and when to do things the right way. I believe you are aware of this because I am aware of it too. It is impossible to get away from it. I have heard people say, "I have no conscience." I do not believe it. I believe they are not paying attention to the voice. They are not heeding the instructions their conscience is giving to them.

36. Be consistent always: It is said that when a person is consistent, life would be easy for such a person. As people are different, so are their behaviors. Some people can be moody, others can be erratic. Ensure your activities are unpredictable. They can be as fascinating as you want them to, but let your behaviour stay consistent towards others. I believe that you have the potential to make your life and that of others better. Remember, there is no point in choosing a path and grow weary of reaching the end.

37. Love life, live life: See the life you are living as a fascinating one. Remember that there are millions - if not billions of people in the world today. Each of them has dreams and aspirations. They are all existing and coexisting in their own way. As long as we are here on this Earth, trying to fulfil a purpose, we must always have it in mind to enjoy life, love life, and live life to the fullest. The only way one can live is by loving life.

Furthermore....

When we talk about the good life, we are talking about a great life worth emulating. Unfortunately, many people find it difficult to find even a slight moment of peace because with so much to do, so much to accomplish, and a lot of obstacles before them, they feel stressed and feel like quitting is the answer. It is not, and for you to enjoy a good life, you need to make your life as simple as possible. This might be difficult for some people to implement but not for you because there are many rules to living a good life, aside the above 30, consider the following:

Tidy and simplify your tasks

I bet you have a lot to do, and when you look at your tasks, it seems harder than you could ever imagine because you have a lot to do within a small period. The best thing to do is relax, tidy up and look for better and simpler ways to handle your tasks. Without this, you would always be stressed out, and you know, stress is not a part of the good life.

Do everything in moderation

For everything that you do, there should be moderation. Just as the popular saying goes, too much of anything is bad. So, everything from TV to eating and even your money spending habit should be done in moderation to avoid unnecessary pressure on you.

Keep your life in perspective

There are times when almost nothing goes as planned, and you find yourself fighting to fix things now and then. One thing you do not know is that we all go through these days as well. All those things you experience would eventually pass, and all you need to do is keep things in perspective. Avoid sweating the small stuff because no matter how difficult it seems; it will eventually pass. All you have to do is keep calm and keep your life and goals in perspective.

Treat others the way you would want to be treated

This is another important rule in life and one which you have to make part of your lifestyle. You need to be sensitive to the needs of others and go out of your way to do something for them. Avoid being judgmental, and try to be nice to people whenever you can.

Have a family first policy

Another path to living the good life is prioritizing your family. No matter what you wish to achieve, you need to know that your family should be a priority. If you choose to work and neglect your family, you will regret that you chose not to spend enough time with them.

Be in the moment

The past was difficult, and the future is unpredictable, and worrying about the past and future can be bad for your health because your past is what it is; your past, and for your future, you can only hope for the best, so your best bet is to be in the moment. Learn to enjoy each day and worry less about what has happened and what is to come. It is then, and only then, you can enjoy your life.

Maintain a positive mindset

If you think negative thoughts all day long, then you would see negative results. However, if you work hard and keep your thoughts positive, you would see good results. It's just the way it works. So, you have to strive to maintain good thoughts because this is the ideal way to live a good life filled with results.

Strive to always learn

The most interesting people are those who always strive to learn every time. They strive to better at everything they do, and this is something people love. So, try to be a lifelong learner, and you would be wise and find people easily directing what they know to you.

Bottom Line

Living a good life is easy; you just need to know what to do to get that life. These rules are not written in stone; they are just a good starting point to getting the good life you have always wanted. No matter where you are, you can always take a bold step to begin from somewhere.

CONCLUSION

"It has been said that time heals all wounds. The truth is that time does not heal anything. It merely passes. It is what we do during the time that helps or hinders the healing process."

Jay Marshall

Life is a journey of many miles, and when you get to the valley, do not quit because it's not the end of the road. Somewhere somehow, you just have to keep on pushing, and the best way to do this is by letting go of all the unnecessary weight holding you down.

One way to do this is to self-heal. In this book, I have covered some of the best ways to heal and become whole as you try to achieve your goals and aspirations. With these tools, you would be able to navigate through difficult times and always come out on top in the end.

You have only one life to live, and you have to make sure that you live that life to the fullest so when you look back at your life when you are old, and of age, you can smile knowing that you lived a happy life free from regrets.

Good Luck.

About the Author

Vincent King a certified psychologist and prolific author who conveys his idea of understanding and compassion in the field of self-help. He has authored numerous self-help books and has touched the lives of many through them. One of his books is "Soul Therapy For The Worried Mind" book which covers various aspects of life that many people are going through at the moment, helping them understand their situation better and guiding them not to give up, but to rather heal themselves.

Vincent is a psychologist, motivational speaker, and life coach. He has used his unique style of teaching to lecture many on the quick way to sound mental well being and to help them out of depression. Many people have recovered from the depression-related and worrying situations, all thanks to his seminars, and books.

He did his Masters programme in Psychology some years back and has practiced as a psychologist for about 5 years. If experience and expertise in self-help is what you need, Vincent King is the right person for you.

www.ingramcontent.com/pod-product-compliance
Lightning Source LLC
Chambersburg PA
CBHW011319080526
44589CB00018B/2734